THE DIET BIBLE

Also by the Author:

Nutrition: The Cancer Answer
Foods That Heal

THE
DIET
BIBLE

The Bible for Dieters

MAUREEN SALAMAN

**Statford Publishing
Incorporated**

Menlo Park, California

3 4 5 6 7 8 9

ISBN 0-913087-03-3

Library of Congress Cataloging-in-Publication Data
Salaman, Maureen Kennedy.
    The Bible diet / Maureen Salaman.
      p.   cm.
    ISBN 0-07-054456-5
    1. Reducing diets.   2. Reducing—Religious aspects—Christianity.
  I. Title.
  RM222.2.S224   1990
  613.2'5—dc20   89-13312
                                                                     CIP

Book design by Mark Bergeron

CONTENTS

DEDICATIONAL

The Book of Books

No wiser book exists in philosophy, in ethics, in human relations . . . counsels for every problem—for bankruptcy, persecution, loneliness, and health of spirit and body. Between the covers of this best seller of all time lie the secrets of success in this world and the next, detailed maps of the road to peace, the passport to eternal life.

Each time I read the Bible, I find the inspiration to guide me, to awaken my mind, to open my heart, to set my soul afire.

Having received such abundant blessing from the Bible, I offer this gift from God to you.

PREFACE

All things work together for good to them that love God. Romans 8:28

I stood on the stage amid the roar of a standing ovation. My speech was over. I felt the electricity in the air, the invisible yet psychically tangible link between speaker and audience that told me I had done more than mouth words—I had touched the spirit of my listeners.

I lead an active life. I travel to interesting places and meet interesting people. There are many whom I admire but no one with whom I would trade places. I like who I am and what I do. But of all my activities there is none so thrilling as that moment at the conclusion of a speech when an audience rises to applaud. This is true not simply because it gratifies the ego (which it certainly does) but because in that moment a speaker feels a special bond with the audience, knowing that their thoughts, their feelings, and their lives have been changed because they have been moved by what was said. Some philosophers contend you cannot move a single grain of sand on the beach without affecting the destiny of the world. How much more fateful is the occasion when you move not a single grain of sand but the spirits and minds of an audience of hundreds or perhaps thousands of people and through them most certainly move the destiny of the world.

When I speak I aim to motivate. I want my audiences to get up and do something about what I have just told them. I want to reach into individuals' lives and change them. It is not enough to inform people. They must be inspired to act. Positive thinking is good. Positive action is better.

But those who have lost hope of achievement are not inclined to positive thinking, nor are they moved to positive action. When I speak about losing weight while restoring health and vitality, I know my words will fall on deaf ears if I do not first impart hope. If people don't believe there is hope of success in what you are asking them to do, they certainly will not even try to do it. They must be made to understand that the lily grows out of the mud. And more than understand it, they must believe it. I can make them believe it because I believe it. And I believe it because I have experienced it in my own life. To paraphrase an old gospel song: "I once was weak, but now am strong; was blind, but now I see."

Of all the pages in this book, the first chapter has been the hardest to write because it is about me. It is hard to write about yourself without sounding either too humble (in an effort to avoid pomposity) or too proud (in an effort to accentuate the positive). Certainly it is impossible to write about yourself without shedding considerable modesty, and you never embark on such a course without the risk that someone else will view the excursion as a display of pure vanity. Yet I think it would be greater vanity for me to propose to direct others along paths that I could not or would not prove that I myself had already traveled successfully.

ACKNOWLEDGMENT

I cannot thank enough James F. Scheer, my collaborator, my editor, my researcher, and, most important, my steadfast friend.

He has devoted wise and patient work to this book.

His reliance on truth, on virtue, and on God is most unfaltering.

If this book is of meaning and help, his is the credit and the praise.

APPRECIATIONS

My deepest appreciation and love flow to Connie and Ronn Haus, of Family Christian Broadcasting Network, who are steadfastly on the course God has mapped out for them. They are a daily inspiration to me to follow more closely the Master's plan for my life.

Their messages are at once modern and ancient—the essence of practicality, because they meet us where we hurt with wise solutions and strong motivations to change. Connie and Ronn are powerful movers of men and women, because their messages follow an unerring path from the Scriptures to the heart.

For Jan and Paul Crouch of Trinity Broadcasting Network. Three little words express my feeling towards Jan and Paul: love, admiration, and gratitude. Well, maybe the words aren't that little, but they are heartfelt. The awesome accomplishments of this duo are shining examples of how, with God, we are an army with whom the "impossible" is "possible."

Starting with abundant faith and little money they were fired up with a vision. Along with their television partners who share their vision, they have built the most far-reaching Christian network in the world, spreading the good news wherever there are eyes to see and ears to listen. I admire them and acknowledge a debt to them. Earlier I mentioned three little words to sum up my feelings for Jan and Paul. Well, some years ago there was a vastly popular song called "Three Little Words." Those three little words also express my sentiments toward them: "I love you."

To two special people in my life: Gene and Karl

Gene Arceri His genius is yet unknown but to a small circle of admirers. But who knows? There is always tomorrow and hope for the renaissance of a nobler time in tomorrow.

Karl Rolfes Whose judgment has been a guiding force for me, as it has the mercurial brightness of pure water.

To those dearest to me: (alphabetized)

Al and Lily Battista Whose courage and commitment to principle make me proud to know them.

Peggy Boyd A beloved person who must take integrity and faith vitamins.

Paul Blumenthal A dear new friend who already seems like a dear old friend.

The Contreras Family My beloved south-of-the-Border medical friends whose staunch idealism and treatment of body, mind, and spirit result in near-miraculous cures.

Gina Foster and Dennis DeLuca Whose lives are committed to honesty and moral truth.

Debbie Fraser Who has benefited thousands with her willing heart and dedication to duty.

Gary Gordon, M.D. Whose innovations not only contributed to the fasting chapters of this book, but distinguished him as one of the great pioneers in the field of natural healing.

Jack Hanley Whose creativity and genius greatly enhanced the quality of this book. It was he who orchestrated the food section.

William Holloway Who gives me hope for tomorrow and hope for America in tomorrow.

Dianna Jackson Who enriches the lives of others with the richness of her own.

Carla Jones With whom I share a rich, comfortable, and old friendship that asks no deeds for reinforcement, nor any deed at all, save that we both stay alive and breathing somewhere like a song.

Stephen Langer, M.D. Who has graciously permitted use of material from his book, *How to Win at Weight Loss*.

Margaret Lesher A friend straight from heaven and masterfully woven into my life by the hand of God.

Dr. Steuart McBirnie A beloved friend who is an army of friends as well as Gibraltar in human form.

Robert Mendelson, M.D. (deceased) The Will Rogers of medicine whose sleight of hand humor remains after him the atomic bomb in our arsenal against medical tyranny.

Dan Ray Who never loses sight of the dream—the American dream itself.

Anne and Jim Regel Who possess that rare gift of being able to go out of themselves and appreciate whatever is noble and loving in others.

Cleo Salinger A woman of beauty on the outside and inside with the serenity of "the still waters" mentioned in the 23rd Psalm.

Dee Simmons Whose dauntless industry and perseverance are the firm foundations of all her many accomplishments.

Glen Simmons Whose unparalleled wisdom, vision, and constant readiness to help are God-given treasures to me.

Jayne Sousa My secretary, my right arm, my right leg, my right everything, an adopted member of my family.

Lee Spellman Whose brilliance can't outshine his personal warmth.

Harold Stueve President of Alta-Dena Dairies, who, in the face of untold persecution, has continued to bring us the finest quality dairy products in the world today.

John Trowbridge, M.D. A giant among medical doctors. His alternative practices of today will be the pattern for the medical profession tomorrow.

Dr. Donald Whitaker Who reached down a hand to pull me up. This is not a self-centered man but a God-centered one.

Holly and Johnathan Wright, M.D. Two great minds and valiant warriors in our noble battle for freedom.

To my son Sean who has inspired me to greater achievements in my effort to be a good example.

To many others whose contributions have found their way either between the covers of this book or in enhancing the lives of others: Cathey and Edward Pinckney, M.D., Irwin Zucker, and my producers, Kathy and John Fitzpatrick.

Theodore Roosevelt once said, "No man is worth his salt who is not ready at all times to risk his body, to risk his well-being, to risk his life in a great cause." Members of the National Health Federation bring this kind of courage to our great organization, and while they are too numerous to name individually, no mention of sacrifice for a great cause would be complete without them: Charlie Fox, Harold Terry, Scott Tipps, Dr. John Trowbridge, Veronica and Fred Niero and the thousands of other NHF members.

My acknowledgments would not be complete without special mention of the following priceless friends: Andrew McNaughton, Dennis Itami, Ron Wright, and Paul Virgin.

CALORIE SECTION

One Pound of Excess Weight

Contains about 3500 calories. To lose that pound, you must consume 3500 fewer calories than your body uses—500 fewer calories per day to lose a pound a week; 1000 fewer calories per day to lose two pounds a week, and so on.

Always bear in mind that weight lost slowly and steadily is more likely to stay lost than weight taken off very quickly.

The Caloric Figures in This Book

Are based on data published by the U.S. Department of Agriculture, or, when specific brands are listed, on data supplied by the manufacturer. All foods that are high in Carnitine are asterisked.

Note Regarding Epigraphs:

Heading each chapter is Scripture which furnishes the acorn from which the oak tree of the chapter grows. Discovering and using these pertinent verses again illustrates to me that the Bible covers every human situation—spiritual, emotional and physical. It comes as no surprise that the Word of God deals with all aspects of human nutrition and even supplies guideposts for stabilizing and losing weight. Let them be your guideposts in the reading as they have been mine in the writing.

When you follow the advice given in this book, you are also following Scripture, so you can't lose—that is, you can't lose anything but weight.

MS

THE DIET BIBLE

CHAPTER ONE

IN THE
BEGINNING . . .

*The waters compassed me about, even to soul: the depth
closed round about me . . .   Jonah 2:5 (KJV)*

*I*NSIDE my trim body was a fat person struggling to escape and
gorge. Sadly, it did—too often. That is why I lost 250 pounds
in ten years.

My weight swings started with five to ten pounds, then rose
to ten to fifteen pounds and up to fifteen to twenty pounds. As
the pendulum swings grew wider, so did my figure—wider and
rounder.

That was the story of my life until I discovered how to melt
off unwanted weight once and for all. Most likely, that is the story
of your life, too—the reason you are reading this book.

My determination to find a solution to my problem began
one morning some years ago when I was at my worst. As I un-
happily surveyed myself—every pound of me—fatigue and
depression, along with my flab, weighed me down.

It was almost inconceivable that only a dozen years before,
I had been a lithe, bouncy, supercharged highschooler who had
won the United States West Coast Cheerleading Championship.

Following that, an energy-draining job as an airline stew-
ardess caused my high-flying lifestyle to take a nose dive. Coffee
and junk food fixes only made me more exhausted. I became such
a chain-drinker of coffee that I jokingly said they should attach
me to a coffee I.V.

I don't know why I went this route, because my mother had brought me up on nutrient-rich foods and supplements: fresh, raw vegetables; brewer's yeast; wheat germ and blackstrap molasses; Tiger's milk; and vitamins and minerals, whose containers seemed to occupy acres of kitchen counter space. My mother had prepared my meals according to the gospels of Gayelord Hauser, Adelle Davis, and Carlton Fredericks.

Coffee, donuts, soft drinks, and diet ice cream were not high enough octane foods for my merciless physical schedule, so I took Dexamil to transform me into an imitation of the lively girl I had once been.

I had "power outs" at 11 A.M. and 4 P.M., as my fatigue and depression worsened. One day while shopping at Safeway, I was so stupefied with exhaustion that I became dizzy and lightheaded and had to abandon my partly filled cart. After following a zigzag path to the haven of my car, I made it home somehow.

Why did my skin no longer glow with the patina and warmth of polished copper? What had become of the vibrant person with a lustrous red-brown mane that gleamed with life and was as strokeable as a cat's fur?

One particularly dark and ominous morning, the gray was so all-pervasive that it seemed to encompass my world and dissolve me in it.

So what did I do to turn things around? I made them worse. I poured a cup of coffee and opened up a convenient package of Sara Lee chocolate fudge cake. Sara Lee had become my patron saint.

Even as I munched this tempting goodie, I knew that Saint Sara Lee would not work the desired miraculous transformation. With the help of God, I had to work that miracle on my own— not only for myself but also for my children.

It was only then that I realized how I had undermined myself and my two children (Sean and Colleen) in nutrition and weight, and the full impact of that realization staggered me. In their infancy, I had slavishly obeyed the pediatrician, who had advised Similac after a year of breast-feeding. As they grew, I fed them canned baby foods, hyped with sugar and salt, as their sole nourishment and then, in later years, cold, sugar-coated breakfast cereal. Was it any wonder they were now hyperactive and over-whelming me with their rebellious conduct?

This guilt trip made me feel even more sickened by what had happened to my body. With grim humor—or was it maso-chism?—I admitted to myself that the sand in my hourglass figure had begun to shift inexorably downward. A shipbuilder could have used a ballast like mine.

I felt that God had played a bad joke on me. It took me some more years of suffering to realize that God had better things to do and that I had been the one who had played a bad joke on myself.

In the midst of my deterioration and my inability to do any-thing about it, I met someone straight from heaven: Helen Sweet, at once my teacher, mentor, and beloved friend. In a world of insecurity and chaos, Helen was order, Divine order. She was a cosmos.

For five years she helped me build the spiritual undergirding that kept me from letting my gloom slide into total despair. A graduate of Moody Bible Institute, she taught me the Scriptures daily.

One day when she was just 59 years of age, she told me the devastating news:

"Maureen, I'm dying of cancer. The doctor says I have only months to live."

I threw myself into caring for her. No one was going to take my spiritual cosmos from me. I drove her for chemotherapy and endured seeing her suffer like a dying animal. She begged to be taken off this treatment, which Hubert Humphrey had called "death in a bottle." Unable to control her bowels and vomiting for six to eight hours daily, she pleaded with her loved ones to jettison the treatment, which was more painful than the actual disease.

"Let me die in peace!" she begged.

Mercifully, the chemotherapy was discontinued. At this point, I began to explore what nutrition might be able to do for her. I was reintroduced to a health food store. I began to fix her fresh carrot juice and to use blackstrap molasses as a sweetener for millet cereal.

Each journey to a health food store was an adventure into a

new land of strange and unfamiliar products. To set a good example for my friend and to give her moral support, I also began to eat this natural food. To my surprise, as I continued to reeducate my junk-food-addicted taste buds, I got a physical and spiritual lift.

I began to feel better. However, in the midst of this triumph, I suffered a devastating defeat. I lost Helen. Although cancer can have a whole complex of causes, I thought often of Helen's case and wondered if it hadn't originated from a poor diet such as the one I had been on. Helen had been faithful to God's word in everything but diet. She had eaten much man-made food instead of natural food. Consequently, she had put on more than a little extra weight.

To get myself and my world back together, I spent some thinking time at beautiful, serene Lake Tahoe. It was there I realized the futility of trying to determine what had caused Helen's death. Probably she had already carried out God's plan for her life. Perhaps it was her time to go.

Late in the day, as I meditated looking into the incredibly clear water, I suddenly understood the power of God. He was the author of all things—the lake, the luxuriant green grass, the shrubs and stately pines on the lake shore, and the stars that made their silvery appearance in the sky as the daylight faded and dusk took over.

It occurred to me clearly that along with my spiritual connection with God, I had to maintain a physical connection through eating food as close as possible to the way God made it. Anything less than that was a compromise that broke my connectedness with God and Godliness.

Somewhere I had read that in fresh, God-made foods the arrangement of each atom and molecule matched the receptors of cells in the digestive tract and thus filled nutritional needs perfectly.

By eating natural God-given food, I would be putting myself back into God's divine plan. My overweight would no longer be a problem. I progressively substituted good eating habits for bad, for example, fresh fruits and vegetables instead of pastries. Then, too, I corrected another error in nutrition. I began again to eat breakfast, which I had omitted for fear of gaining more weight.

Now I made breakfast my main meal, and finally I had the stamina to fix it. To my delight, I lost weight steadily.

There's much more to the story of how I discovered a weight loss formula that has worked not only for me but for hundreds who have followed my simple pattern. This story will unfold in coming chapters. However, the heart of the story is keeping the connectedness through nature to God and through God to nature.

Thanks to my quiet time at Lake Tahoe with God and to my blessed acquaintance with Helen, I have since dedicated my life to learning how to eat for health and wellness—the way God tells us in the Bible—and to show others exactly how it can be done to lose weight and gain health.

As president of the National Health Federation, an organization dedicated to keeping our right to have alternative medicine, editor of *Health Freedom News*, hostess of the worldwide Trinity Broadcasting Network television program, "Maureen Salaman's Accent on Health," and columnist for *Bestways*, a national health magazine, I have interviewed hundreds of natural healing medical doctors, researchers, and biochemists. Their findings harmonize completely with Bible teachings on food and eating, as my in-depth study and searches of the Scriptures reveal.

It is amazing how clear the Bible directions are for abundant health and weight loss. I never fail to be surprised and delighted to find that God cares intimately about what we eat and how our food is prepared.

His Scriptures work for weight loss and wellness. I am living proof of this. Now, at five foot three, I weigh in at 102 pounds and am as slender as I was as a high school cheerleader. My weight is stable; it rarely varies by more than a pound.

At national and regional conventions of the National Health Federation and in my TV fan mail, I am constantly asked, "Maureen, how do you keep your figure so slim? Is there hope for me to do the same?"

Then I tell them that all the secrets—backed by voluminous research studies—are in the Bible. However, most of them say that they don't have the time to do the digging in the Bible and in medical and nutrition journals as I have.

That is exactly why I am committing *The Diet Bible* to paper.

In the process of study, I happened upon a major discovery in nutrition that offers clues to the actual diet for weight loss coming up in the final chapter. Nature never gives us isolated minerals and vitamins. They come packaged in combinations.

We can't comprehend one-thousandth of what still remains unknown in the field of biochemistry.

However, we do know that when we receive these vital combinations from the Master Biochemist, we are obtaining many vitamins that have not as yet been discovered.

It is important to eat God-made food, as opposed to man-made food. Stewards over our agriculture do not use complete fertilizers in preparing the land. They do not follow Biblical injunctions. That is why it is important to grow your own produce if possible, or to buy it from health food stores that guarantee that their products are organically grown. Let me give you a comparison or, rather, a contrast concerning magnesium, which some call the healthful heart mineral. For every milligram of magnesium in a tomato grown with inorganic fertilizer, there are 1938 milligrams in the tomato grown in organically fertilized soil.

Sometimes my TV viewers write in something like, "I don't have much faith in natural organic nutrition."

It is regrettable that most people do nothing to help themselves until nature prods them with a sharp spear of pain or pads them with a gross amount of fat.

My problem—it may be yours, too—was that I was feeding my appetite, not my hunger. I ate what tasted good instead of what was good for me. I ate to eat rather than to nourish myself. I had broken my connectedness with God.

The more vegetables and fruit we eat in their natural state —the way God made them—the closer our diet comes to perfection. (This subject will be covered more extensively in the final two chapters.)

All too many weight loss diets today are crash diets. If we follow them, our health crashes. We can't lose weight properly on a diet so low in amino acids that it cannot feed our body properly. We will be constantly hungry and violate the diet.

It is important to remember that the Bible says that the life of all flesh is in the blood. (Leviticus 17:14, KJV). The building and repairing of the body are done through the medium of the blood, which carries oxygen and nutrients to every living cell. If the body is toxic from junk food, the blood delivers poison to every cell.

Blood has another tremendous task to perform. While building and nourishing are done by the red blood corpuscles, defending the body against harmful organisms and picking up toxins from every organ are handled by the white blood corpuscles, the body's inner army.

Out of my experience and that of others, and from years of study, *The Diet Bible* has emerged. It is easy to follow and rewards you not only in weight loss but also in glowing health and electric energy to supercharge you for your day's activities.

The Diet Bible is as ancient as the Old Testament, yet as new as tomorrow. The Jew and the Christian meet at the dietary laws. [Try the Diet Bible. You'll like it. So will your body!

Then you'll like your body, too!]

CHAPTER TWO

HOW TO SLIM DOWN YOUR FAT MENTALITY

As a man thinketh in his heart, so is he. Proverbs 23:7 (KJV)

"*M*AN is the only animal who eats when he isn't hungry." Mark Twain said it, and he was right on. Eating when you're not hungry springs from having a fat mentality, which causes you to spend a disproportionate amount of time thinking and fantasizing about food. Overweight or obese people think about food not only often but differently.

Whatever your present weight, you will never enjoy healthful slimness without having to work for it. Paradoxically, even inside a slim body—as expressed in chapter 1—there may be lurking a fat mentality lusting to get out and gorge itself.

In order to slim down a fat mentality and the body that can accompany it, you should first know that a fat mentality doesn't come about instantly. It happens by slow degrees as those extra ounces of fat eventually add up to a mountain.

From childhood, you have received a gradual, often subliminal education through the conditioning of 330,000 television food commercials that beguile you and seduce your appetite for food that you don't necessarily need.

So your inordinate preoccupation with things to eat has come courtesy of TV, radio, and the rest of the media, including the slick, colorful women's magazines that feature weight loss diets just a few pages away from recipes for gooey pies and cakes topped with whipped cream.

If it's a question of abstaining from food or indulging in it, the mind always accepts the stronger of the thoughts. The first priority of the would-be weight loser is to mobilize his mentality against excess poundage.

A fat mentality slimmed down by reverse conditioning precedes a slim body. This starts with questioning yourself when you get the compelling urge to eat beyond your needs: Am I really hungry?

Ask your brain, your lungs, your kidneys, your heart, your liver, and the entire range of organs and glands—one by one— Am I really hungry?

You'll begin to realize you're not hungry at all. It's just those years of conditioning that are programming you to home in on the refrigerator. Hunger pangs will pain you for three days. Then they will give way. You will win over your appetite, feel the power of enormous self-esteem, and lose weight. Maxwell Maltz says that 21 days will establish a habit. Hooray for good habit!

The Greeks had a word for what you're doing in reverse conditioning. They called it "repentance." It doesn't mean exactly what most of us believe: being sorry for sins. It means changing your attitude—in this instance, recognizing that extra intakes of food are not necessary. Such extras are what I call "face entertainment."

The more we entertain our face with food, the less entertaining our body will look in the mirror. On the other hand, eating food only for nourishment usually brings quick results in weight loss and exhilaration. You feel closer to your goal and to God.

In interviewing thousands of people who are carrying around tons of extra fat, I find several frequently occurring emotional problems that encourage face entertainment, gluttony, self-pity, bitterness, and guilt.

Are you bitter against any person or life situation? Examine your human relationships and circumstances. Don't gloss over bitterness. This condition not only corrodes the soul, it makes you overeat. Pull out the roots of bitterness.

Then forgive yourself. If you don't do this, you can never

love yourself. It is impossible to obey the injunction of Jesus to "Love thy neighbor as thyself," if you don't love yourself.

Self-pity is actually arrogance. It is similar to saying to yourself, "I'm so great, I deserve to be treated better." As in chain-smoking, you light one sin off another, vindictiveness igniting bitterness.

As for guilt, give yourself a thorough exam to expose your areas of this emotion. Then turn these dark regions of the mind to healing light. Release your guilt, and your feelings of unworthiness will disappear. The Bible has promised that if you confess your sins, God will separate you from them as far as the east is from the west.

Remember, biblical laws work as surely as does the law of gravity. In addition to self-pity, bitterness, and guilt, there is a vast assortment of sins, which, in our subconscious mind, prod us to eat when we are not hungry. Give this emotional garbage away. Let God take it.

Once you do this, just picture yourself as worthy of respect and love. Several BIG women approached me after a lecture on weight loss. BIG is an acronym for *believing in* God. They admitted that when they were young, they were molested by their step-fathers or someone else. Guarding this black secret made them emotionally ill, and their illness made them experience an unnatural, insatiable hunger for food. I urged them to forgive the offender and then forgive themselves, to track each bitterness, one by one, back to the root and forgive and forget it, to give it all to God and leave it there.

They did it, and it is surprising how fast their feelings of self-esteem and worthiness to be loved returned. Almost immediately, they were able to gain control of the appetite that once controlled them.

One of the ways that I mastered my craving for one slice after another of Sara Lee pastries was to acquire the habit of joy. I asked God to let me enjoy the little things in life, to show me how to make them into big things. I call these little joys "tremendous trifles": cherry trees in full pink blossom, a red-headed woodpecker pecking in rivet-gun style on the trunk of a eucalyptus tree, a sunset in full color as only the Master can paint it.

Not only God's natural beauties help me acquire the habit of joy, so do many other things: God in man, a novel observation about our world, or about our bodies and how wonderfully made we are.

It lights my soul with sunshine every time I think of the magnificence of our bodies and minds. Inside them, we have a health kit that can heal cuts, mend broken bones, repair damaged organs, and restore us to healthy positivism and confidence. There is a drugstore inside our bodies that can compound nearly every prescription known to science. Everything to keep our bodies healthy is already within us.

The human body is capable of healing itself of every known disease, provided nothing interferes with its normal function. We act as facilitators in eliminating interferences that occur in these wonderful machines, designed in such infinite perfection.

Every cell has a brain, and it knows if it's to be the iris of an eye, a follicle of hair, or the top of your nose. Your eyes still end up on either side of your nose. Your ears remain on either side of your head. Did you notice you did not have to go to a doctor to grow up? Your body knew how to do it all by itself.

I cannot help reflecting that inside you and me are all the God-given capabilities needed to control our appetites, even if obesity experts now tell us that some of us are programmed to be overweight. We have been given dominion over ourselves by God, so we can reprogram ourselves. It is only hopeless if we think it is. All it takes is sustained faith and patience.

There's fun in giving, in seeing another's face light up at a surprise gift. To some of us, giving is living. And what power there is in these actions to reward us with inner satisfactions so that we don't have to overeat.

What joy there is in laughter.—And there is healing in laughter, as Norman Cousins found.

When I lived for several weeks with the Masai, an African pastoral tribe in Kenya and Tanganyika, to study their health and nutrition, I discovered a happy people who are, for the most part, Christians. Laughter came to them as naturally and unconsciously as breathing their clean, exhilarating air. One of them would touch my lion-colored hair and jump back with uproarious laughter, triggering everybody else's laughter.

I was in awe of these towering, lean, muscular, panther-like Masai. It was as if they were out of another era. Their part of Africa is the primal world. It was like living in the Book of Genesis—a world without walls, without pretense, almost without sound.

There is a special joy in release from emotional negatives of the past—in a new start, a new life, new opportunities. Joy can be found in the little things in life. It is wherever you look for it: in a toddler's first uncertain steps, in mastery of parking a car in a small space, in the quiet patter of rain on the roof to lull you to sleep. The triumphs of family members or friends can also give you a lift for their sake and show you that things impossible are indeed possible, after all.

I observed not one overweight person in the group of several hundred Masais with whom I lived. And how did they remain lean? First, they are far more physically active than we are. Then, too, their preoccupation is with things other than food. These simple, unspoiled people eat Bible foods. In a single day, they consume only as much food as they can hold in cupped hands: maize, lentils, garlic, onions, herbs and fresh vegetables, a small amount of fruit, and on occasion meat from their herds of cows. They drink lots of rich milk.

Never have I seen any people harmonize so well with their environment. They treasure their children and painstakingly teach them tribal lore passed down since the beginning of their history—on taking care of their cattle and living safely with the wild animals all around them. The Masai have always lived amiably with wild animals, with some violent exceptions that come with the territory, as when a tiger invaded their village and killed two tribesmen.

One morning I watched them take their children to the riverside for a nature talk. One of the men showed them the pressed-down grass and, picking up coarse hair, told them that a tiger had slept there and that they should be alert for danger.

For the Masai, teaching is an integral part of living. Each morning they relive the night and rediscover the day, instructing the children about what clues for survival can be found in the remnants of the night. Once a lone black-spotted cheetah darted across the grassy plain after a bulky wildebeest. Too weak to continue the pursuit, the cheetah fell back.

"The cheetah will die," my Masai guide commented. "Today, the cheetah dies and the wildebeest lives. Tomorrow, the wildebeest will die, and the cheetah will live. For everything that dies, something else lives. Jesus Christ died that we might live—eternally," he explained.

After tending their cattle all day—the women and children do most of the milking—the Masai settle down to talk of the day's experiences. Later, they dance with joy, then eat just enough calories as fuel for their myriad activities.

Having traveled to most countries of the world, I have observed that the natives' focus is on things other than food. I was particularly fascinated by the Turks. At four o'clock in the morning during a visit to Istanbul, I heard a clamor beneath my third-floor hotel window and got up to investigate. In the dim, predawn light, dozens of men and boys were gathered in the town square playing soccer. It was all-consuming to them. Everybody wanted to participate.

One incident I observed during the game at first frightened and then impressed me. A 13-year old boy pursued the rolling soccer ball into the path of an oncoming Volkswagen. Hit by the car, he bounded off, retrieved the ball, and kicked the winning goal.

In small towns in Turkey, the natives are so preoccupied with participatory sports and the necessary activities of living—they often walk five miles to a water well—that they have little time for passive activities, particularly compulsive eating.

To the Turks, eating is a necessity, not a recreation. They beat the sun up in the morning, spend the day weaving, making leather sweaters, hand-carving, kneading bread, washing clothes, and carrying blocks of ice for preserving food. They also beat the sun to bed at night.

We have lost the basic concept of food as fuel for activity. Not so the Turks. They often put in three hours of work before they eat. As the Bible states, ". . . If any would not work, neither shall he eat." (Thessalonians 3:10).

Before expert theologians get on my case, I want them to

know this passage is mistranslated but not misapplied by me. Obviously, it refers to those too lazy to work, but it also makes sense looked at from the standpoint of physical activity in relation to weight loss.

Eating should not be a solo activity, as it is with many of us. Eating is a family affair. The Turks maintain a connection with their natural environment; they harmonize with it. Of course, television has found its way to Istanbul and other large cities, but its corrupting influence is not yet widespread.

During a lengthy stay in Turkey, I noted that most Turks do not eat while standing, on the run, or driving a car. Eating is done consciously, not unconsciously and uncontrolled while the eater is under the influence of the television set.

Making a conscious effort to sit down at the table guards you from unconscious eating. Every time I am tempted to stand by the kitchen counter and eat, I visualize Jesus and the apostles standing at my counter and around the sink at the Last Supper.

In Japan too, eating is a special occasion for the family. The ritual of serving is nearly as important as the food. It is almost a disgrace to be obese in Japan, except for the ponderous, blubbery Sumo wrestlers.

In most of the so-called civilized nations, eating is a must when company comes—another excuse for packing away more unneeded calories. The Masai and most of the Japanese have not adopted this habit.

The Masai served us tea but not food. Without the distraction of food preparation and serving, they could give their guests their undivided attention. This is another good reason why there are hardly any overweight individuals among them! It was from them that I mastered the art of listening to guests instead of hearing them without listening.

Another positive force that governs the tendency to overeat is their joy of living and loving. The Masai are loving and affectionate, particularly with their children.

And, finally, there's joy and gratitude and praise for the blessings we receive daily. Again, these blessings do not always come in big packages. Sometimes they are small. However, I have found that by keeping a daily notebook of the pleasant things that have happened to me each day, I am overwhelmed when I review just a month's blessings. Then I can praise God and be thankful for the small and large blessings that come my way.

With a grateful, joyous, loving heart, I am so enchanted by challenges, people, and new things to learn that I rarely think about eating. Sometimes life is so blessed with joy that I forget to eat.

This can happen to you, too. It's just a matter of conditioning yourself in a new way, of focusing on joys other than foods. Then it's easy to diet and lose weight.

And what joy there is in watching those superfluous pounds disappear and seeing a beautiful new YOU appear!

CHAPTER THREE

YOU CAN BEAT THE TEMPTATION TO OVEREAT!

There hath no temptation taken you but such as is common to man: but God is faithful, who will not suffer you to be tempted above that ye are able: but with all the temptation also make a way to escape, that ye may be able to bear it.   I Corinthians 10:13 (KJV)

TEMPTATION to overeat comes in many sizes, shapes, and aromas—often so compelling that avoidance is the first line of defense.

Avoidance is easier than escape, although the latter is sometimes a necessity. You know what foods turn you on and how hard it is to turn yourself off. So avoid freshly baked pastries whose cinnamon aroma tries to seduce you through the nostrils.

Keep your nostrils and the rest of you away from bakeries, donut shops, candy stores, and cookie shops. Plot yourself a temptationless course.

Sometimes temptation is built-in in a place where you just have to go, like the supermarket. The same principal applies: avoidance. Stick to the outer aisles. Those bad goodies that start eating binges are on the inner aisles. Sure, they display candy bars at the checkout counter, but you know where they are and can look away.

Train your eyes to rest only on less inviting foods, not the seductive sweets that trigger binges. One glance at them is enough. The first time you are tempted; the second time you are lost. Why do you suppose restaurants place the tray of French pastries where you can't miss them on the way in? When the dessert cart comes rolling around—hell on wheels—you have been had.

The second ground rule for beating temptation is to flee from it, as the Bible recommends. And as you run, cut off the thought of that chocolate eclair as quickly as a guillotine can descend. The longer an alluring thought makes a home in your mind, the harder it is to evict.

Several studies suggest that you should know thy trigger foods that set off binges—ice cream, cake, candy bars, donuts, or cookies—and never let them into your home. I can almost hear you protest, "Great! But how do I avoid them when I have company?"

You've heard of fresh fruits in season. Nothing is more deluscious. And when they're not in season, use fresh-frozen, sugarless fruits, even though they may not have the high nutrient content of fresh fruits. If your company doesn't go along with something this healthful and low in calories, you may be in the wrong company.

Once you have eaten, put away leftovers. Out of sight, out of mind, and—best of all—out of mouth!

If temptation should overcome you and you go on a binge, don't let one indiscretion destroy your purpose. Forgive yourself and start all over again. It's better to continue striving than to give up.

Everybody wants an easy way to lose weight—a sensational no-diet, no-exercise system that promises to melt away twenty pounds in thirty minutes or less. So everybody jumps on the bandwagon—one bandwagon after another. It turns out that the easy way is the hard way. Wouldn't it have been realistic and easier to go the hard way in the first place?

Speaking of realism, a three-pronged approach works best: diet, exercise, and behavioral modification. This is not just a wild idea of mine. It is based on thousands of interviews with weight losers—some successful—biochemists, and bariatrics specialists (those who treat obesity), and on hundreds of articles on weight reduction in reputable medical, nutrition, and biochemical journals.

Okay, we're all familiar with dieting and exercise, but exactly what is behavioral modification? Changing your way of behaving (living). Unless you alter a lifestyle that brought you the burden of unwanted poundage, you won't win at weight loss. That's basic, no matter what the quick-fix people try to tell you. A new and positive lifestyle means, first of all, changing your mindset about yourself and raising your expectations of what you can accomplish with Divine help.

The chapters that follow will offer you the best fat-melting exercises and the kind of diet that can be followed, including eliminating or at least minimizing junk food. But let's build the program on a rock instead of on sand.

Practice goal orientation. Decide on the number of pounds you want to lose and where. Make it realistic so you won't be discouraged if the fat vacates the place a little slower than you hope. A commercial airline pilot can't very well decide that he'll head the aircraft just anyplace. If he does that, it will be the last "anyplace" he will visit as an airline employee. Likewise, if you decide just to "lose some weight," you won't be too motivated. So be specific, whether it is seven pounds, seventeen, or seventy-seven. This way you'll have a benchmark against which you can compare your progress.

So far as behavioral modification is concerned, you can start with a little realism: "I gained this excess baggage on the installment plan, and it's going to have to leave in the same way."

Let's consider some well-established facts about susceptibility to seduction by food. Heavyweights, more than normal-weights, are turned on by food cues to eat. Also, they are influenced far more by the pleasurable taste to continue eating—that is, to over-eat. Finally, they are more likely to be motivated to eat by food highlighted in stores or wrapped in transparent plastic.

About the point that heavy persons are more drawn to over-eat by pleasurable taste than are normal-weights, a fascinating experiment was conducted some time ago at the Nutrition Clinic of Saint Luke's Hospital in New York City.

Before the experiment was launched, the heavyweights had been averaging some 3500 calories a day, in contrast with the 2200 calories eaten by the normal-weights.

Intake of food for the heavy test subjects was slashed to 2400 calories a day for the first week, then to 1200 calories daily for the following week. The normal-weights were put on a 2400 calorie daily regimen for the same two weeks.

During the third and last week of the experiment, both groups were fed a nearly tasteless, liquid diet enriched with vitamin and mineral supplements to make certain it was nutritionally sound. While the normal-weight test subjects continued eating approximately the same amounts, the heavyweights progressively cut their intake until it averaged only 500 calories a day.

Researchers concluded from this experiment that how much the heavyset eat is indeed more influenced by how pleasurable the taste is than is true for normal-weight persons.

Several other experiments have made the point that heavy people are more turned on to overeat their favorite foods than are normal-weights. They are also more likely to be triggered by outside cues: the hour, the appearance, taste, and aroma of food, and seeing others eating. Knowing these facts can serve as the launching pad for a behavioral modification plan.

Your first line of defense against over-alluring food is at the source—the market where you shop. Food packaging, particularly that of the most harmful junk foods, is so colorful and lifelike that you almost feel the packaging is the product. Madison Avenue seems to know the right combination to reach your susceptibilities.

However, you have the combination for resisting Madison Avenue. Your strength is in knowing your weakness and practicing avoidance. But you can fortify yourself even more with a few hints from weight loss experts. To reduce the urge to buy high-calorie–low-nutrition products, always shop for foods after you have eaten. A full stomach is a staunch ally against temptation.

Several studies substantiate this point. Let's look at results of a representative experiment in which after-dinner shoppers were compared with before-dinner shoppers. The former bought 19.7 percent less food than the latter. When shopping times of both groups were reversed, what happened? The now after-dinner shoppers bought 15.7 percent less food than did the other group.

There's something else you can do to strengthen your resistance—even before you go to the store. Never do freestyle shopping. Always make a list of acceptable foods and never deviate. In other words, it's best to battle temptation on your own turf, with no seductive displays of food products to gang up on you.

One of my friends builds in still more resistance to impulsive, diet-devastating, food shopping. She takes only enough money with her to pay for products on her list.

All right, this business of acceptable foods is fine for an individual or a couple in complete agreement, but what do you do when you must buy for other family members? Simple. As soon as you arrive at home, store the forbidden fruit in the back of your cupboard or refrigerator. This will keep it out of constant sight. Even minor measures like this are effective.

Resisting overeating isn't that difficult. First, eat slowly and chew your food much longer than you normally do. Both practices are helpful in stimulating the flow of throat digestive juices. A friend told me about an interesting finding in this area based on research at the Veterans Administration Medical Center in Minneapolis. This was a study of eating habits of people under stress. A full stomach was not the factor that relieved stress. It was the simple act of chewing.

Individuals who bolt their food feel the necessity to eat again sooner than those who extend the eating process. Many studies show that when you extend your eating to at least twenty minutes, the message of a full stomach has the chance to reach your brain and turn off your desire to eat more. Some people use a timer to see how long it takes them to eat, and many are shocked to learn they're bolting food in ten or twelve minutes.

Many studies reveal that the obese and other heavyweights eat faster than normal-weight persons—another reason why they tend to overeat, particularly the foods they like.

When your day teeters on the brink of becoming an "eata-thon," take a brisk walk so that you burn up calories rather than store them. Another measure I follow when I feel the need is keeping the bathroom scale in the kitchen—as my external conscience. Its presence is a potent reminder of the serious consequences of overeating.

I have never liked certain weight loss programs because you have to record everything you eat. They turn you into a book-keeper. However, keeping a record is an effective move for planning the first week of your weight reduction regimen. Record exactly what foods you ate, the persons with whom you ate, and any factor that contributed to your overeating. This quickie food diary often spotlights triggering foods, persons, places, and incidents—a key to avoiding them.

One of the worst practices for keeping weight in line is eating in front of the television set. I had to learn that the hard way. You are so intrigued with what's happening on the screen that you mouth inordinate amounts of food. Now when I eat, I try to make that all that I do. If you eat unconsciously, you will soon be more than conscious of your thighs and hips.

If you make eating a ceremony, with soft lights and sweet music, and the best china and silverware and freshly cut flowers, by the time you're ready to say grace, you'll be savoring the quality of food rather than the quantity.

You can cut your food intake in many ways. One is to serve smaller portions. If you want to give yourself the illusion that you're still eating as much as before, use smaller plates. Don't ever leave the serving platter parked in front of you. You may be tempted to take seconds or thirds or. . . . Move it right along to some slender person near you. Hosts and hostesses are known for insisting that you have their dessert, especially if it's home-made. Preserve peace in our time. Request a small helping.

You can control the kind of snacks you have at home, so do it. Crunch on carrot sticks or celery, have a heaping tablespoon of cottage cheese, or make do with a small apple.

When the pounds are coming off nicely at one or two a week, give yourself a reward for moving closer to your goal. No, not a food reward. Use what's called positive reinforcement. Congratulate yourself with a nonfood gift: a stereo tape, a book, a new dress or sweater, or a night at the ballet if that's your thing. You know best how to reward yourself.

And while we're on the subject of reinforcement, for two reasons always tell your family and friends you're on a weight loss regimen. You will be less inclined to go off your diet, and you will get some support, along with a lot of kidding.

Another way to cut your caloric intake is not to watch TV before dinner, when every program is punctuated with seductive food commercials. If I'm watching TV with a group at that time,

I simply leave the room when commercials are on. This is a good defensive maneuver, so long as you don't end up at the refrigerator.

Is it hard for you to resist hunger pangs to the extent that you have to fill up on food? Take heart. There are other ways to handle this condition. You can drink a lot of water or tighten your belt.

Probably our faulty eating patterns started in the crib. When baby cries, she is usually fed and gets loving attention at the same time. So subsequent cries may be as much for attention as for food. Rather than eat just because we require food, we eat to satisfy emotional hungers as well. So, as adults we often turn to food when under stress, when lonely, bored, frustrated, unhappy—even when happy—loved, or unloved.

How can you break the iron grip of the past? You simply become analytical, tracking backwards to find your true motivations for eating. You probe to identify and fulfill real hunger for food. When you find an emotional need that powers you into eating, you figure a more direct way of satisfying your emotional need—some low-calorie solution

One surefire method of keeping from overreactive or binge eating is to guard against becoming ravenously hungry. You become too hungry by meal skipping, a subject dealt with in depth in chapter 15.

Another way to avoid giving so much attention to food—and consequently overeating—is to keep busy doing something you enjoy: work, an avocation, or a hobby. Idleness of mind and hands permits vagrant thoughts and imaginings. As Second Corinthians 10:5 says, "Bring every thought into captivity . . ."

If you don't have an absorbing activity, find one. All you need do is give careful thought to this subject. A middle-aged homemaker friend became tired of spending the day eating and gaining her way out of her entire wardrobe. She followed my advice about finding something you like to do and doing it.

As it happens, she had always enjoyed sketching and drawing but had drifted away from it when she got married and began having children. When the children married and moved away from home, she didn't realize she was free to follow her own inclinations.

She submitted some of her sketches to a local ad agency, whose president loved her work and hired her at first part-time and then full-time. Doing something she relished raised her self-esteem and made her feel productive, so she rarely thought about food and within the first several months at the agency lost fourteen pounds and regained her wardrobe.

As with my friend, when you find a hobby, avocation, or career in line with your deepest desires, you won't need incessant food rewards. As a matter of fact, food may slip from first place to second or third.

You may escape temptation this way. But with some individuals, temptation wins, particularly where junk food is concerned. Then they need special armament to deal with the enemy at close hand. This is the subject of the next chapter.

KICK THE JUNK FOOD HABIT— LOSE WEIGHT!

Why spend money on foodstuffs that don't give you strength? Why pay for groceries that don't do you any good? Isaiah 55:2 (LB)

*T*HAT nut-filled chocolate bar in front of you may seem small, but if the temptation to eat it overcomes your will power, it is bigger than you are.

Would you like to know how to resist chocolate, sweet rolls, cakes, pies, ice cream, or salted junk foods like chips and pretzels? Then you came to the right place: the pages of this chapter.

Here's a threefold program calculated to bring you back to connectedness with God and his natural food supply.

1. Create the Right Mental Climate

Use psychological devices on yourself. Imagine the rewards of proper eating: sparkling eyes; clear, flawless skin; a stream-lined, vigorous body; a flat belly; a bright, quick, alert mind; the admiring glance of your spouse or another loved one.

Then as you look at the glazed donuts in the bakery window, you relate them and other pastries to dull eyes; swollen, puffy, pasty, sallow skin; an always exhausted, bloated body shaped like a sack of meal; and a dull mind characterized by power outs, anxiety, fatigue, and depression.

Every time you see some junk food, just associate it with the negative qualities it helps to cause. Reread the paragraph above so that you can visualize these negatives.

Look at a brown sausage and a slice of white bread. The sausage is made from undesirable animal parts and laced with the harmful chemicals nitrate and nitrite; the white bread is baked from devitaminized, demineralized, and chemicalized white flour. Consider them as brown and white death because they are not live foods. Review the thought that dead foods produce death.

═══════════ 2. Reinforce Yourself ═══════════

Read articles and books about the benefits of natural, live foods. Listen to radio and TV programs that reinforce your stance on eating healthful foods, as well as reinforce your backbone. Understand that cravings come about not just from an empty stomach but mainly from low blood sugar and food sensitivities and allergies, and that today's foodless foods create the need for eating, eating, EATING!

Remember the Bible Scripture, "And ye shall eat and not be satisfied." (Leviticus 26:26, KJV). Also recall the old Bible quotation that is as new as this minute:

"Why spend money on foodstuffs that don't give strength?
Why pay for groceries that don't do you any good?" (Isaiah 55:2, LB.)

Visit your local nutrition center and get a liberal education. Learn to avoid foods grown with synthetic rather than organic fertilizers and with pesticides, herbicides, and fungicides. Buy whole grain breads and cereals. Take in all the nutrients God put into them, not just those that food processors left behind.

Examine the advertising double-talk that enriched white bread is nourishing. It may be nourishing compared with its wrapper. Then, again, it may not be. Likewise, sugary breakfast foods are ideal for sharply raising, then sharply lowering, your blood sugar, for increasing your food cravings, for helping you stay overweight and assisting you in developing dental cavities or caries—the latter is the more popular term. Who ever heard of popular cavities?

Researcher William H. Philpott, M.D., has found that eating embalmed, processed food almost devoid of enzymes is a major cause of diabetes. The pancreas can't synthesize enough enzymes to make up for this dietary deficiency.

Like other processed food, sugar has a specific deficiency— no vitamin B-1—and therefore has to draw upon what little is available in the body. Sugar cane and beets come with sufficient vitamin B-1, but makers of table sugar refine it away. When you eat considerable amounts of sugar and fail to take a B-1 supplement, pyruvic acid cannot be converted to a helpful nutrient and thus, along with lactic acid, is believed to contribute to rapid heartbeat and eventually to an enlarged and waterlogged heart.

Other systemic sabotage caused by refined sugar (refined flour, too) is loading the bloodstream with glucose, which encourages reactive hypoglycemia, a condition in which blood sugar soon plummets to often dangerous levels. Usually, the junk food eater munches a candy bar or cookie to restore a proper level and give himself a new shot of energy.

But then comes the severe drop again, and with additional highly refined carbohydrate fixes, the up and down swings become even more pronounced. You suffer fatigue, hopelessness, and the blues, and you are ever hungry and keep eating more empty food and adding more poundage.

My friend William Campbell-Douglass, M.D., of Marietta, Georgia, warns his patients against eating processed and imitation food products. His pet admonition is, "If man made it, don't eat it!"

Imitation milk and artificial creamers are examples of dietary no-no's. (For more information on them, see chapter 5, "Imitation Foods for Real People.")

3. Keep From Craving

As touched upon earlier, low blood sugar triggers cravings for food, and refined carbohydrates ensure a seesaw blood sugar level reflected in energy highs and lows. You can stabilize the seesaw by eating whole grains and raw vegetables in place of junk foods.

Coffee, hot chocolate, caffeinated soft drinks, and nonherbal teas also contribute to low blood sugar (hypoglycemia), particularly coffee with its high caffeine content.

Coffee jolts the adrenal glands to release adrenalin, which revs up the tempo of the entire glandular symphony, increases blood sugar, and in turn stimulates the pancreas to secrete insulin, which then lowers the blood sugar level. Again, you have the seesaw pattern, hypoglycemia, and cravings for another food fix.

Substitute fresh vegetable juices for coffee and "chew" them so that your mouth enzymes have a chance to work, or drink herb tea or spring water with a dash of lemon.

Fresh, raw vegetables are excellent for bulking the stomach, giving that full feeling that kills appetite, and for supplying fiber for regularity and vitamins, minerals, and coenzymes for metabolizing these foods.

Though not generally considered junk, the apparently innocent items served by fast-food establishments fall into this category because of the way they are prepared.

Chicken and fish, recommended by the National Heart Association as low-fat items to replace beef, are in most instances fried in beef tallow—trimmings from meat rendered into shortening. Tallow is high in saturated fatty acids, said by many authorities to raise blood cholesterol.

Potatoes are french-fried in the same superhot, bubbling tallow solution, which occasionally contains some vegetable oils, too. Fish nuggets were found in a *Science Digest* survey to be dripping with beef fat—37 to 40 percent saturated fat. A chicken sandwich in one fast-food chain contained 42 grams of beef fat. That adds up to as much fat as is found in a pint and a half of ice cream.

Fat that you're not told about is what I call "sneaky fat." Various fast-food chains have replaced tallow fat with vegetable oil for frying fish nuggets and chicken, but they have retained beef fat for french fries. Authorities on fast foods say the best beef tallow is used because it gives food a unique flavor.

Fast foods—maybe we should call them "fat foods"—may

be hurrying their eaters into an early grave or at least into overweight, because, as chapter 7, "Go Easy on Fat Foods," shows, a diet heavy in fat leads to an accumulation of fat in the human body. So slow down on fast foods. Better yet, cut them out.

It is estimated that a typical fast-food meal—a double burger with cheese, sauces, and french fries—gives you 67 grams of fat, not far from the average person's daily fat intake of 89 grams.

Fat-rich foods contribute not only to overweight but also to cardiovascular disease and cancer. Therefore, it's best to make a quick getaway from fast foods.

Although it's not difficult for most individuals to desist from eating an extra hamburger and another order of french fries, it's not easy to shake repeated seduction by sugary foods. Usually, the three recommendations made earlier in this chapter will work. However, if candy, sweet rolls, cookies, cake, and sugared drinks still remain bigger than your will power, you may wish to consider the surefire system of Abram Hoffer, M.D., of Victoria, British Columbia, for cutting them down to size.

His procedure works because it is based on God-given reflexes present in human beings since the beginning of time. Surrounded by thousands of plants, most of them poisonous, the earth's inhabitants discovered food that wouldn't kill them. How did they and the animals manage this?

Dr. Hoffer answers with an illustration: If you feed a wild rat enough poison to make him sick but not kill him, the rat will not eat the poison again. He explains, "The rat has learned that it ate something which made it bring up, and, therefore is not going to touch it one more time. . . . If you feed a coyote lamb meat laced with lithium, which will make the animal very sick, that animal will no longer eat lamb meat."

According to Dr. Hoffer, "A motion picture was made of a coyote that had been made sick this way. After he had recovered, a small lamb was placed in front of him. The coyote took one look at the lamb, vomited, and ran away. This is a natural conditioned reflex in all mammals—an aversion toward foods that make them sick."

If sugar and sugared products are so harmful for us, then why don't we all develop an aversion to them?

We don't for two reasons: They taste good (taste doesn't warn us as poison did the coyote), and we are conditioned to sugar from infancy (in baby foods), when our dietary intake is out of our control and in the hands of mothers and grandmothers who force sweets on us.

Says Dr. Hoffer: "We gradually become sick of these sweets but don't have a chance to develop the aversion reaction. If you're trying to train adults not to eat this junk, you have to show them that they'll get sick when they do eat it."

Parents needing advice from Dr. Hoffer about helping their children quit eating junk foods are told to keep them from sugar or sugared products for six days.

"I declare Saturday to be Junk Day," he explains. "So the children are very pleased that on Saturday they can have all the junk food they want."

Openly Dr. Hoffer tells the children he is permitting them junk food because he wants them to get sick and to feel the effects of that sickness.

"On the seventh day, they eat ice cream and chocolate bars with coke for breakfast, again for lunch, and again for dinner. The mother is instructed to shove it in until they're screaming with pain," explains Dr. Hoffer.

This may seem an extreme, even cruel, treatment, but children who have made themselves sick in this way soon stop eating junk, according to Dr. Hoffer. Usually just one Junk Day is necessary to make the point.

"Let me give you a practical example," he says. "A mother with seven children brought two of them to see me. Both were hyperactive. One of the children was a very good, cooperative patient, the kind every doctor loves. He stayed away from sweets completely after I asked him to. When the mother came back a month later, he was normal.

"The second child refused to cooperate. His mother couldn't keep him away from sweets, and when I saw him a month later, he was no better.

"So then I advised the mother that she ought to try this technique. The following Saturday the mother started the two children. She wanted even the one who was refraining from sweets to try it.

"Upon her declaration of Saturday as Junk Day, the other

five children became very much annoyed because they were being deprived of this fantastically nice day. The mother said, 'Okay, you can all have it.'

"So all seven children went on the junk all day. By nightfall, they were vomiting. Half of them had migraine headaches. Some were so sick they could hardly move. That did it. A month later, the little, bad boy came to see me. He was fine and relaxed, doing well. I asked:

'How do you like that junk? Are you going to have any more?'

" 'No,' he replied. 'I'll never touch that stuff again.' "

Unfortunately, children aren't the only ones who eat excessive amounts of junk food and suffer the cumulative ill effects, including weight gain. Dr. Hoffer notes this phenomenon in adults, too, particularly through the Christmas holidays. January becomes the adults' relapse month, when patients come to him with depression, headaches, migraine, and tension. They ask if the holiday cakes, cookies, and candy caused these symptoms.

"Yes," Dr. Hoffer responds, and then encourages them, saying, "I'm glad you did that. It's very important that you make yourself sick regularly so that you'll understand how important it is that you keep away from sugar."

Numerous heavyweight or obese individuals I have known have tried Dr. Hoffer's method of breaking the addiction to sweets. Every one of them has been succesful.

Should you want to try it, you must first desist from sweets for six days so that your body can be cleared of them. This is necessary so that when you take in a large amount of sugar, you become very sick. Dr. Hoffer likens his procedure to a tolerance test for a food sensitivity or allergy. It doesn't work in every case but is effective in most instances.

Hoffer cautions that adults and all parents must be judicious as to whether they should have a Junk Day for themselves or their children.

Another warning should be issued. In the instance of severe hypoglycemia, diabetes, or any other serious disorder, a junk food program could be hazardous to health and even to survival. Consult your family doctor before you try it.

Queried about the possible hazards of his program, Dr. Hoffer responds:

"Is there danger of getting too much sugar? Not as much as the danger of chronic overdose that you're going to give yourself for the rest of your life if you're not taken off it.

"None of my patients has been harmed by a Junk Day. As a rule, as soon as they get thoroughly sick, they don't eat the stuff anymore."

And isn't that the reason for Junk Day?

Eliminating junk food from your diet, no matter how you manage to do it, is a major step toward mastering your weight problem and reducing poundage so that you can become the person you want to be.

CHAPTER FIVE

IMITATION FOODS FOR REAL PEOPLE

. . . And ye shall eat and not be satisfied. Leviticus
26:26 (KJV)

*A*WISE friend and candid observer of the human scene recently told me:

"With people consuming so many imitation foods and
beverages—among them synthetic eggs, cheese, milk, coffee cream,
dessert topping, ice cream, and fruit drinks—it's a wonder they
don't turn into imitation people."

In a sense, they do!

A diet high in man-made food—for weight loss or anything
else—and nutrient-impoverished, highly processed, canned and
packaged products almost assures a person that his health will
deteriorate to a mere imitation of what it could be.

I am sad that so many weight reduction diets include junk
foods, many of which are supposed to help us escape from a high
cholesterol regimen—but don't, as you will soon see.

These nearly foodless foods separate us from nutrient-rich
gifts from God and from God himself. They break our connectedness to Him. Each of these dietary deceivers is a colossal pre-
sumption, telling God that He didn't know how to do the job
right—a massive monument to man's arrogance.

Seeing imitation and/or processed foods in weight loss diets,
I am especially distressed, because within a severely limited num-

ber of calories, no one can afford to eat nutrient-deficient foods. A friend who has been around to eat God's great food for longer than I have tells me that the late syndicated columnist, William Brady, M.D., had an appropriate name for these counterfeits: "cheat foods."

As you will see a few pages from here, Dr. Brady was right on! For the defense of the body in which God delivered you into the world, it is important to know the truth, for the truth shall set you free from cheat foods and from overweight, marginal health or illness, and a needlessly shortened life.

Even today's so-called genuine foods are not what they appear to be. Like Hollywood films, they are only the illusion of reality. And illusions are not noted for their food value.

I'm talking about steadily declining amounts of protein, vitamins, and minerals in fruits, vegetables, and grains as reported by authorities on soils. Just as inflation is subtly and insidiously eroding the dollar, so are some major agribusinesses depleting soils and, along with them, your health of body and mind.

Evidence of this is disclosed in extensive studies by the late William A. Albrecht, Ph. D., chairman of the Department of Soils at the University of Missouri, and from official government reports.

As revealed in congressional testimony, five-ingredient chemical fertilizers do not begin to replace numerous trace elements taken from the soil by crops. This is like being overdrawn at the bank, depositing $5000 and writing a check for $100,000. It won't work too well. (More about this later.)

Between the good earth—actually, the not-so-good earth—and your gullet, crops lose many nutrients in harvesting, transporting, canning, or freezing. Consequent shortchanging of proteins, vitamins, minerals, and enzymes invites degenerative diseases with their attendant misery and, pertinent to our subject, gnawing, abnormal hunger and a powerful drive to overeat.

Let's get back to first things first: imitation foods for real people.

One of the factors driving people to imitation foods is the superscare campaign put on about fat- and cholesterol-containing foods. In later chapters I will talk more about the fact that blood serum cholesterol can be lowered in many natural ways (at least eleven) other than eliminating some of the good foods, although I do advocate cutting down on fats in ways noted in chapter 10.

In any event, imitation foods, for which the receptors of our trillions of cells were not created, are not as easily assimilated and made available as the ones provided by God. And if they are not as absorbable, we get another subtle deduction of nutritional values, which makes our cells cry out for more and more food even when the stomach is full.

Remember the Bible verse at the head of this chapter: "And ye shall eat and not be satisfied." That's the story of imitation foods and natural foods grown in impoverished soils.

One of the most distressing aspects of imitation foods is that sales propaganda has fooled consumers into thinking that the imitation is as nourishing as the real.

A recent poll by the Food Marketing Institute reveals the "don't care" attitude of consumers, even when the bottom line is their health, survival, and—unknown to them—their ability to stay on a diet.

Just 50 percent of the consumers queried were concerned about the nutritional content of their foods. This represents a decline of 10 percent over the previous year. What price trust and indifference!

Want to know what consumer priorities were? Not nutritional content. Only less salt, fat, and cholesterol, and fewer calories. The "phony phoods" industry pushes freshness, homemade taste, no matter by what potentially health-sabotaging chemical the taste has been implanted, pretty colors, lower cost (this doesn't always hold true), and convenience foods.

The latter should really be called "inconvenience" foods because the time saved in preparing them is dwarfed later by the time spent in pharmacies, doctors' offices, and hospitals because of them.

Let's get into some of the main reasons for this—major product by major product—starting with margarine, which your favorite physician probably told you is the equivalent of butter but contains less cholesterol. (I touch upon this aspect briefly in chapter 10, referring to margarine as a tragic joke to biochemists.) Several surveys disclose that many people think that margarine is better for you than butter, mainly because of the cholesterol issue.

Supposedly it has a lower content of fat, which is purportedly unsaturated. This is false, inasmuch as both butter and margarine contain about same amount of fat and both are saturated. Vegetable oils used to make margarine take up oxygen readily and become rancid quickly, so they are infused with hydrogen (hydrogenated) to keep their freshness. By this process, they actually become saturated.

Some years ago a flood of promotion about the merits of polyunsaturated oil and margarine for preventing cardiovascular problems inundated physicians. Swept along by the propaganda, doctors began recommending polyunsaturated oils and margarine to patients (many still do) unaware of two hazards: 1) an increase of these oils in the diet can cause premature aging, encourage certain forms of cancer, high blood pressure, liver damage, and blood sludging (abnormal clotting of red blood cells); and 2) hydrogenated oils, with a higher melting point than butter, can't be as well utilized by the body, don't circulate in blood or through tissues in liquid form, and may clog cell membranes, blocking nutrients from flowing into and out of cells.

Experiments with animals and human beings by Dr. Hugh Sinclair at the Laboratory of Human Nutrition, Oxford University, revealed that hydrogenation of fats causes a deficiency of essential fatty acids. The results? Arthritis, atherosclerosis, cataract, cancer, neurological disease, and skin ailments.

Franklin Bicknell, M.D., a distinguished British scientist, explains the reason for Dr. Sinclair's findings. Hydrogenation rearranges the atoms of essential fatty acids (EFA) from the way God arranged them, and therefore the body cannot utilize them. Further, these atoms prevent the use of normal forms of EFA. They contribute to a deficiency, therefore, even where there is a sufficient supply.

In an experiment by Dr. Fred Kummerow, professor of food chemistry at the University of Illinois, nine groups of twelve pigs each were fed balanced rations with 3 percent fat represented by beef tallow, corn oil, butterfat, fat and sugar, egg yolks, crystalline cholesterol (equivalent to that in two eggs), or other fats.

One group was given a diet high in hydrogenated fat. Fifty-eight percent of the pigs in this group developed raised lesions of the aorta, a first stage of hardening of the arteries. This figure compares with just 14 percent in all other groups.

So much for the benefits of margarine.

Now for imitation eggs, such as Egg Beaters, laid by chemists. Their advertisers call them a cholesterol-free egg substitute. Actually, a substitute is supposed to be a replacement, the implication being that the replacement has qualities similar to the original.

Ersatz eggs are usually low in phosphorus and manganese, minerals in which the good egg is high, and lacking usable or bioavailable sulfur, vitamin A, niacin, zinc, and additional trace minerals.

Beatrice Trum Hunter, in the *Great Nutrition Robbery*, states that the synthetic egg mixture has almost ten times as much sugar and starches as the genuine egg. Diabetics should be aware of this. She also writes that there is 133 percent more sodium in the artificial egg than in a real, large egg, a fact those on a low sodium diet should know.

Like artificial eggs, imitation cheeses are made from a hodge-podge of products: a compound of casein—the milk protein in natural cheese—with calcium, potassium, or sodium, usually highly saturated coconut oil, vegetable oils, hydrolyzed cereal solids, protein, color, flavoring, and salt.

These low-cholesterol products that taste and look like real cheese are advertised to food retailers as having a shelf life of about a year. That is, they won't develop mold before that time.

This is fine for food processors and supermarkets, but what about you and me? Biochemists tell me that high biological quality is often based on how quickly such a product will develop mold.

Dr. Elmer V. McCollum, former professor of biochemistry at Johns Hopkins University, recommends, "Eat only foods that rot, spoil, or decay—but eat them before they do." On this basis, so far as the value of a food goes, shelf life is really shelf death.

Another synthetic product worth mentioning, but not worth drinking in place of milk, is imitation milk made mainly from soluble soy protein. Polyunsaturated fatty acids are added, presenting the specter of an overabundance of them in the diet and the possibility of premature aging along with the other goodies mentioned earlier. The fat in some imitation or filled milk is saturated and hydrogenated coconut oil.

If man-made milk is supposedly the equivalent of what emerges from Bossy or Elsie, why does it have only one-fourth to one-ninth of the calcium and only one-third to one-quarter of the phosphorus?

Although cow's milk has a reasonable degree of uniformity of vitamin content, depending on caliber of feed, imitation milk does not. Some of it contains no vitamin A, in which real milk is rich; others have token amounts. Most brands of ersatz milk have no vitamin B-2 and are low in protein.

Beatrice Trum Hunter states that by unanimous agreement of researchers, imitation milk has been declared not suitable for infants and children and "potentially harmful" for pregnant and lactating women, persons on marginal diets (low-income groups), and the aged.

If you think that nondairy creamers for your coffee and cereals are lower in fat and more healthful than real milk or cream, forget it. Their principal ingredient is either coconut oil or palm kernel oil, two of the most saturated fats. They are loaded with sweetening agents (sugar and corn syrup) and an arsenal of chemicals, many not intended to invade the human body.

The same is true for substitutes for whipping cream and whipped toppings. If you use these products and want to experience fear of the unknown, read the lengthy list of forbidding ingredients on the labels.

If you like imitation ice cream, the following will come just in time to ruin your dessert course. Most brands boast that they contain no butterfat. True. They replace it with animal fats such as tallow and various oils—coconut (highly saturated), corn, peanut, soy, and/or cottonseed oil. Then, too, there are goodies such as sweeteners—making up about 16 percent of the content—emulsifiers, and stabilizers.

Now hear this! Imitation ice creams that use cottonseed oil get a special and unwelcome ingredient that is not listed on the carton. Because it is not essentially a food crop, cotton is literally drenched with pesticides, which concentrate in the oil.

The story on synthetic fruit drinks is not quite as frightening, except that buyers—particularly young people—are led to believe that the artificial is the real and therefore as nourishing.

Ersatz orange juice pretty much tells the story of all synthetic juices. Processors of imitation juices trumpet the information that their brand contains more vitamin C than real orange juice, which may be accurate. But there's a great deal of difference between the bioavailability of natural vitamin C in fruits and vegetables and that in the synthetic vitamin C thrown into imitation orange juice.

Additionally, real O.J. contains some Vitamin B-1 and niacin—usually omitted from imitation juices—and four times as much potassium, as well as other minerals, trace minerals, vitamins, bioflavonoids, and fiber. God created these nutrients in oranges for His own reasons without the added sugar, artificial colors, and flavors of synthetic orange juice.

Some years ago the processors of an orangeless orange drink called Tang boasted in advertising that the astronauts took their product to the moon with them. Perhaps they should have left it there.

On the desk before me is a news story from the Center for Science in the Public Interest (CSPI), a Washington, D.C.-based consumer protection organization. They surveyed brand-name fruit beverages and found that they contain anywhere from 5 to 50 percent real fruit juice.

Do you suppose the labels of these diluted products tell you what percentage of real fruit juice you're getting? You know the answer to that. CSPI revealed that some of the diluted products —I call them "the liberally water-baptized"—sell for more money than the 100 percent pure juices.

CSPI mentions that at this writing the Food and Drug Administration (FDA) proposes to rescind a regulation (little observed or done so in microscopic type) requiring fruit beverage producers to disclose on labels the percentage of real juice in their drinks.

Hey, FDA, supported by our tax dollars, whose side are you on?

As man loses connectedness to God—the vertical relationship—he loses connectedness with man—the horizontal relationship—and thinks in terms of his own self-centered interests and benefits.

This is how whole grains were almost processed out of their nutritional value. Several generations ago, only whole grains were sold to consumers. However, grains could not be shipped long distances without spoilage, which cost processors profits. Then about 100 years ago, the high-speed roller mill was invented. This separated out the nutritious parts of the grain, the germ and bran. These were fed to hogs, and the rest was reserved for human beings.

That's how anemic white flour was born, with twenty vitamins and key minerals missing. From it came anemic white bread. And so the staff of life became a broken crutch.

Public pressure brought on the alleged bread enrichment program, in which twenty milled-away nutrients were replaced with three vitamins and two minerals. Enrichment could more rightly have been characterized as "de-impoverishment."

Heavily sugared breakfast foods, also de-impoverished, addict children to sweets and can contribute to dental caries, hypoglycemia, diabetes, and obesity. Some of these products also offer such special nutritional benefits as "snap, crackle and pop." And their shelf life is incredible. Eat enough of them and you'll be on the shelf longer than the products.

When I attend nutrition conventions, I keep hearing the old standard about breakfast foods being less nutritious than the packages containing them. Supposedly, as a joke, researchers at a western university performed an experiment with rats: One group was fed the sugar-laden cereal and the other the cartons in which it came. You guessed it, the latter group came out healthier.

Contrary to conditions in the breakfast food industry, processors of certain products do their best to serve you the maximum nutritional values: canners and freezers of vegetables or fruits. Despite their best intentions, however, too many nutrients are lost.

This is why I do not recommend canned or frozen foods in *The Diet Bible*. They must all be fresh. Long years of experience have taught me to use vegetables and fruits right from the garden if possible. The reason? I get the benefit of the enzymes, which spark or speed up biochemical processes.

If you don't or can't have your own organic garden, buy your vegetables or fruits from a farm-fresh produce market or right from the farm, and refrigerate them immediately to slow down enzymatic action. Enzymes decompose in fresh foods and cause rapid loss of nutrients. It is best to eat vegetables raw, lightly cooked, or stir-fried.

Although preferable to canned, fresh-frozen vegetables lose trace minerals due to the use of chelating agents in the processing. Also, salt and sugar are often added to them.

Let's look at typical losses in our foods. Dr. Richard Passwater, a prominent biochemist, states that peas taken right from your garden lose 56 percent of their vitamins in cooking. Fresh-frozen peas take an 83 percent deduction of food values in processing: scalding, freezing, thawing, and cooking. Almost all the vitamins in peas—94 percent—are lost in the various steps in canning: scalding, sterilization, liquor diffusion, and reheating.

Many weight reduction diets shortchange you nutritionally, because their nutrient values are less than realistic. Customarily, food values of raw products are used as a measuring stick, from which 25 percent is deducted as the calculated loss from exposure to light, oxygen, and high temperatures, and from storage and shipping. On a weight reduction diet including canned, frozen, and otherwise processed food, food value losses are far greater.

At the beginning of this chapter, I mentioned a basic problem of our food supply: depleted crops from depleted soils. Why is this so? Vegetables, fruits, grains, and legumes have no special ability to draw more nutrients from the soil than are in it.

Five-ingredient chemical fertilizers cannot replace the numerous trace minerals that have been drawn out of the soil by a long succession of crops. Even magicians have to put a rabbit into the hat beforehand to be able to draw it out later.

Food values of most crops are steadily declining. Although you appear to be getting the same products year in and year out, you are actually paying far more for far less, even without considering inflationary food prices.

Earlier the late Dr. William A. Albrecht, an authority on soils, was mentioned in connection with studies of declining soil fertility. One of the problems he noted is the diminishing ability of crops grown in poor soil to synthesize protein.

Albrecht found that over a ten-year period, the amount of

protein in alfalfa and corn had declined from 9.5 to 8.5 percent. Certain amino acids that are usually present had disappeared.

The same thing is happening to wheat, he reported, adding that some diseases of human beings can be considered traceable to deficiencies of trace minerals in soil.

God made us stewards of the earth to have dominion over all things: plants, animals, birds, and the living things in rivers, lakes, and oceans. With that stewardship came connectedness to God and responsibility.

In a statement reminiscent of the Bible's reminder of our stewardship, Albrecht points out that we are at the top of the biotic pyramid, supported down the ladder by plants and animals and then microbes and soil. Likewise, they are dependent on us. Our inferior stewardship has led to neglect of the soil through incomplete fertilization and consequently to neglect of the other members of the biotic pyramid from the ground up to us. As a result, our biotic pyramid partners are neglecting us. We are the only pyramid members who can correct the situation.

Albrecht continues, saying that plants can make carbohydrates quickly from air, rain, and sunshine with only a minor assist from the soil. Thus crops pile up bulk. However, to synthesize protein, crops need help from a fertile soil. He decries the little-recognized fact that soil can be quickly raped of its protein-producing power, although its carbohydrate-making capacity will continue long afterward.

Numerous research studies by the U.S. Department of Agriculture, the University of Illinois, and the Alabama Agriculture Experiment Station verify the Albrecht findings, demonstrating the necessity for proper fertilization to maintain correct production of protein in relation to carbohydrates. (Declining protein in vegetables, fruits, and grains is bad news for those who try reducing weight through strict vegetarian and fruitarian diets.)

Other documentation about soil neglect comes from the testimony of Allan Cott, M.D., before the Senate Select Committee on Nutrition and Human Needs. He told members that to support life, soils must be fertilized completely, not fractionally, with all needed trace minerals.

For more than a century, certain soils have been cultivated only with the conventional fertilizer containing just nitrate, phosphate, potash, calcium, and magnesium. Therefore, the plants and animals that we eat are, like the soils, deficient in trace minerals.

Speaking before the same committee, Michael Lesser, M.D., cited government reports stating that the soils of thirty-two states lack zinc and that the commercial fertilizers contain none of this mineral.

Another multiphase problem with agricultural giants farming vast acreages is so all-encompassing that it deserves a book in itself, so it can be covered only superficially here. I'm talking about unbalancing the ecology with pesticides, herbicides, and fungicides.

Yes, I know about the necessity for feeding a starving world population and the argument that "you can't do that without insecticides." But the world is full of good minds that can come up with ecologically nondestructive solutions to the problem.

Many years ago, shortly before his death, I spoke to Francis M. Pottenger, Jr., M.D., one of the rare foresighted medical doctors at the time who knew that "food is our best medicine" and pioneered nutrition for patients and anyone else who would listen. His name is kept alive today in the name of an organization championing the same cause: The Price-Pottenger Foundation.

Dr. Pottenger told me that insect problems became magnified when farmers did away with hedgerows and windbreak trees between farm properties. "Birds roosting there fed on insects and protected crops. Further, you protect the food supply by selecting the hardiest seeds and complete fertilizers. Healthy and well-fed plants resist insects and diseases."

Not long ago, I had as a guest on my TV program Ken Anderson, who lectures nationally on health, nutrition, and ecology. Ken drew a flood of laudatory letters from viewers. He stressed subjects related to the ideas of Dr. Pottenger, for example, the need to get back to hardy seeds instead of the present hybrids. The hybrids produce greater yields per acre of less nutritious foods that leave us more hungry, and they do not reproduce themselves, he explained.

In June 1987 a *Reader's Digest* article similar to my discussion with Ken, "SOS—Save Our Seeds!", by Lowell Ponte, explained the vulnerability of hybrid crops to blights and wholesale insect attack. One of many laudable things mentioned in this article was encouraging work of the Seed Savers Exchange for collecting and sharing superhardy, prolific heirloom seeds that grow great vegetables, fruits, and grains.

Using such seeds, passed down through the generations, could bring about a rebirth of agriculture. If you want to contribute to a problem's solution, here's how to contact the organization, headed by Diane and Kent Whealy:

Seed Savers Exchange
R.R. 3
Box 239-D
Decorah, Iowa 52101

While agreeing with the *Reader's Digest* article, Ken Anderson went on to explain another constructive step being taken by some farmers to upgrade the quality, food value, and insect-resistance of crops that is particularly suited to small acreages. In line with Dr. Pottenger's observation about the need for birds as a way to control insects, he said that new agricultural research has shown that plants respond to morning bird calls by opening up cells to receive the dew on leaves and blossoms. Experiments have shown that bird calls transmitted by a sound system that covers as much as twenty acres of crops makes the plants more receptive to dew. When nutrients are sprayed on the plants and the morning bird calls are transmitted, plants grow almost to double their size and contain two or more times the nutrients.

Here's another worthy idea for farmers—particularly small farmers—to consider. Farmers near cities could experience a revival of their fortunes if they grew crops organically, advertised the fact, and sold them to a burgeoning population of enlightened people through roadside stands and local health food stores. The retailers could use suppliers of fruits, vegetables, and eggs from chickens raised on the ground and not given growth hormones and shot full of antibiotics.

These are a few ideas to put into your computer. And from my observations on a worldwide basis, they compute. It's time to renew our stewardship of the land, to regain connectedness with God, and to supply and eat sound foodstuff that promotes radiant health and a reducing diet that we can live with. As it stands, most diets are something we can live without.

CHOLESTEROL, WEIGHT LOSS, AND YOU

And he took butter and milk and the calf which he had dressed, and set it before them; and he stood by the tree, and they did eat . . .   Genesis 18:8 (KJV)

*W*ATCH your cholesterol!
Don't eat eggs! Don't eat butter! Don't drink whole milk!

Let me add one more "don't" to the list. Don't go by the above "don'ts"! All we have drummed into us today is to avoid cardiovascular disease by cutting down on high-fat, high-cholesterol foods. Is this good sense, nonsense, or somewhere in between?

As the verse above shows, butter, milk, and meat were eaten by people in the Bible. These foods and eggs are God-given foods. However, in various chapters of the Bible, we are told to practice moderation, not deprivation.

Although there are differences of opinion on the subject, many solidly grounded authorities assert that only the small fraction of the population afflicted with hypercholesterolemia—one in 500 persons—must omit fat- and cholesterol-rich foods entirely.

Further, we have several built-in protective mechanisms against too much cholesterol. The liver and individual cells shut off production when there is no shortage of it, and the intestinal wall has a limited capacity to absorb cholesterol and permit it to enter the bloodstream. So most excess cholesterol just passes through.

Are the authorities who rabidly insist that everyone should

go on a low-fat, low-cholesterol diet on a solid base or are they off base?

We've all heard the medical establishment's position, including its insistence some years ago that we add polyunsaturated oils to our diets. It quietly retreated from this position when research showed the harm excessive intake of polyunsaturates can cause—premature aging, liver damage, lung deterioration, degeneration of the reproductive organs, and breast cancer, among the major disorders.

How about equal time for the other side of the issue, not only to reveal that there *is* another side but also to show that some of God's good foods from biblical times to today are being arbitrarily eliminated from diets for no sound reason.

Has a clear-cut case been established for the low-fat, low-cholesterol diet being crammed down the throats of Americans? Does it really help anyone other than the miniscule number of hypercholesterolemics?

Dr. Stewart Wolf, of the University of Texas, and Dr. John Bruhn, of the University of Oklahoma Medical School, addressed that very question by analyzing more than one hundred medical articles on the claimed risk factors in heart disease, in an attempt to isolate a common denominator in diet that could justifiably be named a risk factor in heart attacks.

These articles, from various nations of the world, revealed not a clue to any particular fat that could be branded a cardiovascular culprit. Nor could the two researchers find that blood cholesterol level had any particular effect on heart disease.

When proponents of the low-fat, low-cholesterol diet find themselves running out of ammo to defend their position, they reach way back in time, stating that heart attacks decreased drastically in Europe during World War II because high-cholesterol foods were scarce.

It so happens that that illustration holds about as much water as a fish net. Broda Barnes, M.D., Ph.D., checked into this matter in depth, spending many a summer in Graz, Austria, poring over the most complete and detailed autopsy records in the world. He states:

"Certainly high-cholesterol, high-fat foods were scarce during World War II in Europe. Certainly heart attacks did decrease, but investigators didn't consider all phases of the issue in depth and came to the wrong conclusion.

"Rather than make a thorough check of autopsies, they made the error of counting only the number of persons who died of heart attacks."

Over a number of years, Dr. Barnes studied autopsies recorded between 1930 and 1970 to learn the truth of the issue. In order to benefit the living, he went to the dead, 70,000 of them.

In the war years between 1939 and 1945, heart attacks indeed dropped sharply. But unexpected evidence almost jumped off the records at him. In no way had the low-fat diet protected arteries from atherosclerosis!

The number of persons under fifty with atherosclerosis had actually doubled between 1939 and 1945, and the damage to the arteries of these individuals was almost twice as great on a scale of zero to four. The low-cholesterol diet had not protected the arteries at all, because atherosclerosis had multiplied by four times.

"At first I was mystified," Dr. Barnes admitted. "Then I discovered that deaths from tuberculosis had risen much faster than those from heart attacks and understood why. Tuberculosis patients usually don't live beyond forty years. This was not quite long enough to have heart attacks.

"In almost every case, patients who died of TB manifested greatly damaged coronary arteries. If adult patients had not died of TB, they would have been cut down by a heart attack within a short time. Wartime conditions had replaced heart attacks with tuberculosis as the major cause of death. A low-cholesterol diet had had not a thing to do with protecting people from heart attacks.

"A few years after that, everything reversed," Dr. Barnes observes. "Antibiotics became available, saved the lives of tuberculosis patients, and deaths from heart attacks rose. The autopsies revealed the truth. Adults dying from heart attack showed healing tuberculosis in the lungs. Antibiotics which had stopped immediate death from TB had given the chance for advanced arterial damage to become the killer."

If the low-fat, low-cholesterol diet is such a winner, how come so many high-fat diets of various nations seem to have no influence on blood cholesterol level? Let's take a look at a study of the diets of residents of Roseto, Pennsylvania, reported in the *Journal of the American Medical Association*, and similar studies of Somali camel herdsmen, the Masai tribe of Tanganyika, and Cook Islands natives.

Low-cholesterol devotees would be horrified by the typical Roseto diet, which appears to be all "no-nos": numerous eggs, fatty meats, many foods fried in lard, and other high-cholesterol delights such as prosciutto ham ringed by at least a half-inch of saturated fat and peppers fried in lard.

On this diet, which seems a shortcut to suicide, citizens of Roseto had cholesterol levels like that of the rest of the nation: 136 to 500, averaging 224. But wouldn't a diet this outrageous cause cardiovascular carnage? An eleven-year study revealed a negligible number of heart attacks in under-55-year-old Roseto men. In those over 65 who showed evidence of heart disease, there was a high survival rate.

Now for the Somali herdsmen, who usually drink five quarts of high-fat camel milk each day. Wouldn't you think their blood cholesterol would be out of sight? Not so. The highest reading recorded was 153.

As I mentioned earlier, the Masai tribe lives mainly on milk—its fat content is twice that of ours—the grain they can hold in two cupped hands, and some meat. Their average cholesterol level? Just 125. Heart disease is almost unheard of to them. Over-65-year-old natives who were autopsied after accidental death manifested inconsequential atherosclerosis.

Two groups of Polynesians on the Cook Islands in the South Pacific were compared on the basis of diet and number of heart attacks. One group ate little saturated fat; however, the other ate twelve times as much. Heart attacks were virtually absent in both groups.

Several recent studies seem to link elevated cholesterol more securely with cardiovascular disorders. Most authorities affirm that blood cholesterol levels above 220 should be reduced. The medical orthodoxy, with its strong orientation toward drugs and medicines, favors drugs when or if the low-fat, low-cholesterol diet doesn't work, and often it doesn't.

There's a major problem with cholesterol-lowering drugs: devastating side effects. Granted, in life or death conditions there may be justification for taking the risk of anti-cholesterol drugs. But this is a matter between you and your doctor. In most instances, however, cholesterol can be lowered by natural means without taking away foods that are essential to abundant good health, weight loss, and longevity.

If you need guidance in any of the following eleven surefire methods for lowering cholesterol, you can find a preventive medicine specialist or a wholistic doctor in your area. Any nutrition center (health food center) can direct you to one.

Here are the Big Eleven:

1. Munching three raw carrots daily. (The crunching will either drive others in the room nuts or force them to join you in self-defense.)
2. Following a vegetarian diet. (Also include eggs and dairy products if you're not allergic to them.)
3. Eating four or five bowls of cooked oat bran each week.
4. Pursuing a high-fiber diet.
5. Taking a pectin supplement each day.
6. Adding a lecithin supplement to your regular diet.
7. Eliminating added sugar and sugar-laden foods from your diet.
8. Supplementing your regimen with 1000 milligrams of vitamin C daily.
9. Correcting low thyroid function.
10. Making sound adjustments to the stresses of life.
11. Doing regular and vigorous aerobic exercises daily.

1. Munching Three Raw Carrots Daily

Almost a certain winner for reducing cholesterol levels, this Peter Rabbit fare offers fiber and bulk, filling your stomach so that you won't be so prone to overeat and go off your diet. Carrot eating doesn't have the risk of strict vegetarianism since it is a supplement to the daily diet, and a nonfattening supplement at that.

=========== *2. Following a Vegetarian Diet* ===========

A great many studies, usually by the Seventh Day Adventist group, have shown the effectiveness of the vegetarian diet in reducing cholesterol levels and maintaining such lowered levels. Vegetarianism also elevates levels of HDL, the favorable form of cholesterol, and lowers LDL, the unfavorable form.

Almost every biochemist I know professionally and personally favors the less strict kind of vegetarianism, that is, one that includes eggs and dairy products. This eliminates the danger that there will be insufficient vitamin B-12 and vitamin A and zinc in your diet.

An element of risk always accompanies long-term vegetarianism: pernicious anemia from insufficient vitamin B-12, which is present in vegetables and fruit only in a negligible amount.

Luke Bucci, Ph.D., formerly chief biochemist at the M. V. Anderson Hospital in Houston and now in the same capacity with Biotics, Inc., tells me:

"We need only an infinitesimal amount of vitamin B-12 daily, but we have to make sure we get that or take the chance of developing pernicious anemia, which can cause disturbances of the nervous system, brain deficiency, and even death.

"Even as a biochemist, I would not pursue a strict vegetarian diet. I would take the insurance of eggs and dairy products. For the benefit of those who enjoy Russian Roulette, there is a warning signal of impending pernicious anemia. The tongue and mouth begin to burn, but this could be caused just as readily by lack of hydrochloric acid in the stomach as by insufficient vitamin B-12."

Dr. Bucci mentions also that strict vegetarians should take a vitamin B-12 supplement to augment their diet, preferably a brand that includes what is called "the intrinsic factor," which makes this difficult member of the B vitamin family more readily assimilated.

Many vegetarians are deficient in vitamin A—a fact they are not usually aware of—because of faulty liver function or hypothyroidism (low thyroid function). Sometimes hypothyroidism is at the root of faulty liver function, too. Carotene, the vitamin A precursor, cannot be translated into vitamin A unless the liver is working properly. Insufficient thyroid hormones in the blood can also block carotene translation into vitamin A.

Dr. Luke Bucci additionally recommends 10,000 I.U. (international units) daily of vitamin A supplement for vegetarians who refuse to add dairy products and eggs to their diet.

Without sufficient vitamin A, the thyroid gland cannot efficiently take up iodine, its principal food, and its function is therefore weakened. Also, the pituitary gland, the quarterback of the glandular team, degenerates without sufficient vitamin A and cannot produce enough thyroid-stimulating hormone, which is the quarterback's signal to the thyroid to run with the ball.

In addition to the possible shortages of vitamins in strict vegetarianism there is the possibility of insufficient zinc. In the previous chapter it was mentioned that the soils of thirty-two states are zinc-deficient. So, consequently, are the vegetables and fruits grown in them. For this reason, Dr. Bucci recommends a daily zinc supplement of milligrams.

3. Eating Four or Five Bowls of Cooked Bran Each Week

Several studies have shown that four or five bowls of cooked oat bran a week can definitely lower your cholesterol. A further advantage is that it produces less gas than wheat bran.

My friend Jeffrey Bland, Ph.D., a biochemist of note, says that just seven tablespoons of oat bran consumed daily can reduce a person's blood cholesterol by 13 percent or more. That could mean a drop of twenty to thirty points for many individuals, enough to take them out of what is considered by some authorities as the danger zone: anything above 220.

Jeff advises that people sprinkle three or four tablespoons of uncooked oat bran on other breakfast food, add it to batter of baked food, or mix it with fruit or vegetable juice or milk.

4. Pursuing a High-Fiber Diet

For many years, clinicians have known that fiber helps lower blood serum cholesterol level. However, it took the investigation of Denis Burkitt, M.D., a public service health physician of South Africa, to dramatize this fact for the world through an in-depth, 10-year study of dietary fiber in relation to coronary heart disease, cancer, and other degenerative diseases.

In the study men who ate the least fiber had the highest mortality rate from coronary heart disease—four times greater than that for individuals who consumed the most fiber. Then, too, the rate of death from cancer was three times higher among the low-fiber eaters.

The conclusion of the study was that at least 37 grams of fiber daily—about seven tablespoons—protect us from coronary heart disease, cancer, and other degenerative disorders.

Remember that fiber is obtained not only from grains but also from fruit, vegetables, legumes (beans and peas), and nuts.

5. Taking a Pectin Supplement Daily

By taking a pectin supplement daily, you can add another inner ally to your defense against excessive blood serum cholesterol. Just what is pectin? Without it, jelly wouldn't jell. Pectin is that gelatinous stuff that helps jelly get it all together and stay solidified.

Rutgers University researchers assert that pectin helps lower cholesterol, and in this way contributes to preventing heart disease. Their theory is that pectin governs the amount of cholesterol the body can absorb.

Dr. Ancel Keys, a distinguished pioneer in cardiovascular research, and his associates at the University of Minnesota conducted a controlled experiment that revealed that pectin did indeed make small but distinguishable reductions in blood serum cholesterol level. When the pectin supplement was discontinued, the level rose to its previous height.

6. Adding a Lecithin Supplement to Your Regular Diet

For more than a generation lecithin, an oily substance derived from soybeans and in recent years from eggs, has been lowering blood cholesterol in numerous experiments. Initially, such favorable results were pooh-poohed by the medical establishment and the Food and Drug Administration as only they can pooh-pooh.

In recent years, however, the negative reaction has diminished, the result of a special report for the Food and Drug Administration by the Life Sciences Research Office of the Federation of American Societies for Experimental Biology.

Citing a long list of lecithin triumphs, among them enhancing memory and cognition, the report enumerated cardiovascular benefits such as lowering triglycerides (blood fats) and cholesterol. And—get this—lecithin actually reversed deposition of cholesterol on walls of arteries.

Scientists at the Simon Stevin Research Institute in Bruges, Belgium, conducted an exciting experiment in which 100 patients were given lecithin for fourteen days. The patients manifested an average decline in blood serum cholesterol level of 40 percent.

Another experiment, this one by Dr. Lester Morrison, who formulated the initial low-fat, anti-cholesterol diet, demonstrated that the Belgian results were not a happenstance. On a supplement of six tablespoons of soy lecithin daily, twelve of fifteen patients found that their blood cholesterol had declined by an average of 41 percent.

7. Eliminating Added Sugar and Sugar-Laden Foods

A study by the USDA's Human Nutrition Center demonstrated that certain individuals, particularly men, can't metabolize carbohydrates (sugars and starches) and consequently their blood levels of cholesterol and triglycerides rise along with their levels of insulin.

In the late 1950s USDA experiments showed that a decrease in the intake of sugar significantly lowered blood cholesterol levels in lab animals.

In 1957 John Yudkin, professor of physiology at Queen Elizabeth College of London University, released results of a fifteen-nation study of coronary disease in relation to the average intake of sugar. Annual deaths from coronary disease per 100,000 individuals skyrockets from 60 for a yearly sugar intake of 20 pounds to 300 for 120 pounds annually, and then spikes into outer space with 750 deaths for 150 pounds of sugar per year.

A lot of other such evidence exists, and has for many years. Many researchers think that sugar intake is more damaging than fat intake. Of course, sugar producers are not too keen about the word getting out. After all, they are trying to protect their bottom line.

To sum it up, eating added sugar and sugar-laden foods regularly could spell sweet suicide.

8. Supplementing Your Regime With 1000 MG of Vitamin C Daily

As Dr. Linus Pauling has long held, vitamin C can reduce the risk of heart disease. It is actually a triple threat because it: 1) lowers total blood cholesterol; 2) decreases triglycerides and LDL cholesterol (the harmful cholesterol), and 3) increases HDL, the good-guy cholesterol.

Dr. Pauling cites research by Dr. Emil Ginter, chief of biochemistry at the Institute of Nutritional Research in Bratislava, Czechoslovakia, showing that vitamin C regulates total blood cholesterol: increases the rate at which cholesterol is taken from the blood and converted into bile acids and then excreted with the bile into the intestines. Taken before breakfast, vitamin C exerts a laxative effect and hurries waste material through the bowel, lessening the chance that bile acids will be reabsorbed and converted into cholesterol.

Constance Spittle, M.D., a well-known English pathologist, experimented on herself regarding vitamin C relative to cholesterol level. She began taking 1000 milligrams of vitamin C daily. Within three months her cholesterol reading had dropped to 130. Her next step was to introduce this practice to fifty human subjects. Every one of them taking this daily amount of vitamin C showed a drastic reduction of blood cholesterol!

====== *9. Correcting Low Thyroid Function* ======

In a later chapter we mention hypothyroidism (low thyroid function) as one of the impediments to losing weight. Hypothyroidism can also be an impediment to lowering cholesterol.

Much hidden hypothyroidism exists because blood tests for this disorder are specific for the ailment but not always sensitive enough to detect it. This is why the Barnes Basal Temperature Test (the armpit test, to be detailed later) is so important. IT IS ACCURATE. If you find you are hypothyroid, you can almost be certain your blood cholesterol level is higher than it has to be.

Orthodox medicine does not accept the Barnes Test. To the establishment, it has objectionable features: it costs the patient nothing; it eliminates an expensive lab test that is not accurate enough but which doctors believe in; and, worst of all, it is not new. If a drug, technique, or piece of diagnostic equipment isn't the latest thing, it is too old, and so the wheel must be reinvented. So what if it's square? Not remembering history, or ignoring it, the medical profession must relive it.

In the early 1930s abundant medical research existed to show a clear-cut relationship between low thyroid function and elevated cholesterol, but such information is too old to be new.

Way back then, a study by a physiologist named L.M. Hurxthal revealed high blood cholesterol in hypothyroids and low cholesterol in hyperthyroids. Two other researchers of that period found elevated cholesterol and blood fats to be symptomatic of hypothyroidism and that a give-and-take relationship exists between the decrease in basal metabolism in thyroid deficiency and the rise in blood cholesterol. In fact, this relationship is so precise that they had a mathematical formula to describe it: The rise in cholesterol is four times as great as the drop in metabolism.

Dr. Broda Barnes has told me that iodine in the food supplement kelp can often correct the underfunction of the thyroid gland in first-generation hypothyroids, but that the actual thyroid hormone, prescribed by a doctor, is needed to compensate for this condition in patients of second-generation hypothyroids or beyond.

"With kelp or thyroid hormone, the patient usually experiences an appreciable drop in blood levels of cholesterol and fat," comments Stephen Langer, M.D., of Berkeley, California, a thyroid authority.

10. *Making Sound Adjustments to the Stresses of Life*

Inasmuch as it's impossible to avoid all the stresses of life, we have to develop a pattern for coping with them. Whatever pattern that is will determine whether or not our cholesterol and blood fat levels soar or remain relatively stable. (More about that in chapter 13, "Don't Let Stress Sabotage Your Diet!") Improper reaction to mild or moderate stress can cause us to overeat.

Several adjustments that can be made over a period of time for better coping are adopting a cheerful, positive outlook; dedication to work; feeling in control of your situation; and building stamina. Any vigorous, sustained aerobic exercise can also bring stress relief and fend off overeating.

11. *Doing Regular, Vigorous Aerobic Exercises Daily*

Several well-structured experiments have demonstrated that daily, vigorous aerobic exercise not only lowers the harmful LDL cholesterol but increases HDL, the good cholesterol. Among the notable experiments is one conducted by Josef Patsch and associates at the Baylor College of Medicine.

Various physical activities do the job: jogging, brisk walking for thirty or more minutes at a stretch, hiking, folk dancing, swimming, and tennis.

Patsch warns that there's no quick fix. Benefits continue for very little time after the exercise program stops. He suggests building time into your lifestyle for daily exercise and continuing for the rest of your life.

The same goes for understanding your nutritional requirements and for planning, preparing, and also following a food regimen that's right for you.

GO EASY ON FAT FOODS

It should be a perpetual statute for your generations through all your dwellings that ye shall eat neither fat nor blood. Leviticus 3:17 (KJV)

REMEMBER the fairy tale about Jack Sprat who could eat no fat and his wife who could eat no lean? Remember the physical consequences of their diets?

Jack ended up with a spare figure, and his wife ended up with a figure to spare.

Biochemically, the story of the Sprats is no fairy tale. It's too true to life. A diet heavy in fats can make you obese even if the calories consumed are moderate.

Rat experiments conducted by University of Illinois, Chicago, researchers reveal that high-fat diets of the same calorie count as low-fat diets lead to high-fat eaters weighing 32 percent more. Their carcasses were 51 percent fat, compared with 30 percent for the control group. The obese rats became that way without actually overeating, say biochemists Lawrence B. Oscai, Margaret M. Brown, and Wayne C. Miller.

Three groups of rats had access to all the food they wanted to eat, their diets ranging from 42 to 50 and 60 percent fat content. The fourth, control group's diet contained approximately the same number of calories but just 11 percent fat.

So much for fat rats. Do these illuminating findings pertain to human beings? According to Miller, yes. A typical U.S. diet contains 40 or more percent fat, and the biochemical principles involved are similar in animal and human. Miller indicates that reducing that percentage of fat could be an important key to weight loss.

Another pointed question is why the same number of calories would cause different degrees of obesity. Aren't calories the critical consideration? All the returns aren't in as yet, but the University of Illinois researchers discovered that rats on a high-fat diet metabolize fat differently from those on a more moderate diet. There are enzymatic changes that the researchers are now trying to understand.

Judging from research conducted by Dr. Eliot Danforth, Jr., professor of medicine at the University of Vermont, the same biochemical principles apply to human beings. In one experiment a group of adult men was overfed a diet of mixed fat and carbohydrates, while another group was overfed a high-fat diet of fewer calories. You guessed right. The fat eaters gained thirty pounds over twice as fast as those on the mixed diet—in less than three months compared with seven months.

Why? Danforth has found that in the process of storing fat from the two classifications of food, 23 percent of the carbohydrate calories are burned off contrasted with only 3 percent of the fat calories.

Confirming the Danforth experiments, Dr. J.P. Platt, professor of biochemistry at the University of Massachusetts Medical School, states that most of the fat stored in all the old familiar places comes from fat in the diet.

Furthermore, it is essential for heavyweights and normal-weights who wish to burn off excess pounds to realize a central fact about the major food classifications, carbohydrates, fat, and protein. So far as calorie content is concerned, all classes of foods are not created equal. (Thank you, President Lincoln!) One gram of fat contains nine calories whereas one gram of carbohydrates or protein contains four calories.

Are the findings of this research the reason God told his people not to eat fat, as the Scripture at the head of this chapter orders? And does this mean we aren't supposed to drink whole milk, use cream, or eat butter or cook with it?

Not at all. God was referring to animal fat such as that of the ram, which was part of the sacrificial offering to Him, as stated in Exodus 29:22 (LB). Reserved exclusively for Him were ". . . the fat tail, the fat that covers the insides, the gall bladder and the kidneys and the fat surrounding them . . ."

Now we are living in times of hysteria about cholesterol. There is a wildfire epidemic of "cholesterolphobia." Establishment medicine warns that we must cut our intake of foods containing large amounts of cholesterol and fat, almost eliminating God-given, nutrient-rich foods such as meat, milk, eggs, and butter.

Is this wise or otherwise?

Otherwise. First, because when these so-called authorities deprive us of these necessary, life-giving foods, they are violating Bible scripture, and second, because when they offer no comparable food substitutes for the bald reason that there are none, they are shortchanging us nutritionally. Yet, these individuals feel so secure in their stainless steel cocoon of self-righteousness that they are unaware of the inevitably devastating physical consequences they are building into the futures of misguided millions who blindly follow their dictates.

Most frightening now is a propaganda campaign advocating that everybody from two years on up be tested for blood serum cholesterol level, and that those above a certain figure be put on this low-fat, low-cholesterol diet and possibly even be treated with drugs to reduce blood cholesterol. Many pediatricians I know, even some in official medical organization positions, are horrified at the very thought of this happening, for the rock-solid reason that developing children need fat. So do we all, for that matter, although not as much as most of us are getting.

This campaign uses scare talk about eating meat, milk, eggs, and butter. It wants us to substitute fish for meat. In moderation, this is not a bad thought, but it, too, has its drawbacks. They say we should substitute low-fat or nonfat milk for whole milk, imitation eggs for the real things, and margarine or polyunsaturated oils for butter.

Let's compare these manipulations of man, these health fads, with the Word of God.

In Timothy 4, the first five verses, we are alerted to the perils of the latter times and the danger of departing from the faith under the influence of "seducing spirits and doctrines of devils" and "speaking lies in hypocrisy forbidding to marry and commanding to abstain from meats, which God hath created to be received with thanksgiving . . ."

If milk were harmful, God would not have referred so enthusiastically to "a land flowing with milk and honey" in so many books of the Bible: in Exodus (four times), Leviticus, Numbers, Deuteronomy, Joshua, and Jeremiah, among others.

If God had wanted it any other way, He would have referred to his Promised Land as "the land of low-fat milk and refined sugar." Eggs are mentioned in various parts of the Scriptures, and it is common knowledge that they were eaten in Old and New Testament times when available.

So far as butter is concerned, the prophet Isaiah revealed it to be a favored food in these words: "Butter and honey shall he eat, that he may know to refuse the evil and choose the good." (Isaiah 7:15, KJV).

Instead of being allowed to eat God's good, natural foods in peace, we are being assailed with ill-founded propaganda that they are harmful even in moderation—propaganda contrary to the Scriptures.

The anti-meat faction makes the valid point that today's meat comes from cattle deliberately confined in claustrophobic feedlots to be fattened for market, rather than from active, range animals as in former times. However, meat in moderation is a healthy and strength-building food.

(Then, too, animals are given hormones and antibiotics, an unwelcome adulteration. The same can be said about poultry, with the exception of that sold in health food stores and in certain kosher meat markets. Health food store beef and lamb are also free of hormones and antibiotics. Little known to the general public is the fact that some fish are also treated with antibiotics.)

You may be surprised at the following information about meat. Edward R. Pinckney, M.D., former associate editor of the *Journal of the American Medical Association* and an in-depth researcher of cholesterol for many decades, states in *The Cholesterol Controversy*, written with Cathey Pinckney, that studies reveal that meat fats show little if any effect on blood serum cholesterol level.

The Pinckneys refer to other experiments disclosing the startling fact that beef and many other meats contain no more cholesterol than the same weight of fish fillets.

Of course, ocean fish contain a polyunsaturated oil that is protective against heart attacks and also fatty acids called Omega-3: eicosapentaenoic acid (EPA) and docosahexanoic acid (DHA), which lower blood fat (triglycerides), increase the proportion of good cholesterol (HDL) to harmful cholesterol (LDL), and reduce the danger of abnormal blood clotting that can cause heart attacks and strokes.

Not long ago there was a justifiably big flap when a certain watchdog of the food industry announced that fast-food chains were deceiving the public by deep-frying fish fillets in beef tallow, a saturated fat, mainly because it made the product taste better.

The attitude of the fast-food chains seemed to be: Forget about health; taste is the thing. In response to this revelation, most of the chains changed over to polyunsaturated oils. What an improvement! When polyunsaturated oils are heated, they become more saturated. This is not just an irresponsible, unfounded observation. It is a documented, direct admission of the former chairman of the Excutive Committee of the National Safflower Council and a top executive of a major vegetable oil company.

In *The Cholesterol Controversy*, the Pinckneys write: "When a polyunsaturated fat or oil is heated, there is a chemical action that causes the polyunsaturate to act with the oxygen in the air and form a polymer or a new chemical compound that is usually the same chemical multiplied manyfold.

"Plastics are polymers. Varnish and shellac are polymers. In fact, it is the heating of polyunsaturated oil that produces varnish. That polyunsaturates form varnish in the body was demonstrated when animals fed such heated fats were found the next morning stuck to their cage floors by their varnish feces. Some of the animals suffered total intestinal obstruction from the polymerized polyunsaturates.

"When animals were fed heated polyunsaturates and heated butter to note the effect on their health, the animals fed the heated corn oil had markedly lower growth rates, developed diarrhea and their fur became rough. All the animals given heated corn oil developed tumors, and only one of the original 96 survived the 40 month experimental period. In contrast, none of the animals fed heated butter developed tumors and all survived.

"When a polyunsaturate is heated, it acquires a new, lower iodine number. The iodine number is the way fats are determined to be saturated or unsaturated. The lower the number, the more saturated the fat is supposed to be. Thus, cooking polyunsaturates lowers their iodine number and, therefore, they could be thought of as more saturated, another fact which seems to be ignored by those promoting cooking with polyunsaturates as a preventive or cure for heart disease."

A finding about polyunsaturates never brought to public attention by the medical establishment was revealed by Dr. David Kritchevsky, of the Wistar Institute in Philadelphia, Pennsylvania.

One of his experiments demonstrated that corn oil heated for just fifteen minutes before being fed to animals actually enhanced atherosclerosis. The longer polyunsaturates are heated and reheated, the more hazardous they become to the health. Think this over the next time you order deep-fried foods. The oil your french fries are sizzling in may be old enough to be eligible for Social Security.

Sadly, I admit that the West Germans are more progressive than we are in this matter. A food establishment owner who reuses cooking oil for more than three days is imprisoned and given a stiff fine.

Frightening results of animal and human experiments would make any knowledgeable person avoid deep-fried foods, particularly when eating out. Female animals fed heated corn oil had an increase of 127 percent in breast cancer. Similar animals fed heated butter showed no increase in cancer, and the latter outlived the former.

When Dr. Roslyn Alfin-Slater of UCLA fed heated polyunsaturates to lab animals their reproductive capacity was impaired. A diet of 10 percent or slightly more of heated polyunsaturates fed to animals by Dr. A.L. Tappel of the University of California at Davis caused testicle damage when heavily concentrated in that area. In a similar experiment the lab animals' diet was made up of 15 percent polyunsaturated oil, and every animal died within three weeks.

Dr. Denham Harman, professor of medicine and biochemistry at the University of Nebraska and an authority on longevity, deplores the excessive use of polyunsaturated oils because various studies of animals and human beings show that these oils bring on premature aging and actually shorten the lifespan.

A two-year experiment by Dr. Pinckney with Dr. Cadvan Griffiths, a prominent Beverly Hills plastic surgeon, was conducted to determine what if any effect polyunsaturates voluntarily added by patients to their diet for cardiovascular protection had on characteristics of their facial skin. The dietary practices and physical appearance of 1012 subjects were reviewed by an impartial third-party professional.

Each patient was evaluated according to these major criteria: the degree, depth, and number of wrinkles—frown lines, crow's feet, and monkey lines—and skin flabbiness or firmness, color, elasticity, and resilience. Allowances were made for excessive exposure to X-ray or sun, for dentures, and for water retention as exhibited by swollen eyes in the morning and swollen ankles at night.

A minimum of 78 percent of the patients who admitted being on a diet of more than 10 percent polyunsaturates displayed obvious signs of premature aging, as observed in facial features by the third-party plastic surgeon. Many of them appeared to be more than 20 years older than they were. Let's hear Dr. Pinckney's summation:

"When this group was compared to an almost equal number of those who made no special effort to eat polyunsaturates, the difference was profound. Only 18 percent of the latter group were judged to have outward physical signs of premature aging.

"In other words, there were more than four times as many people who looked markedly older than they really were in the group that intentionally stressed large quantities of polyunsaturates in their diet."

One of the funniest—or most tragic—inner-circle jokes among biochemists is the common belief that margarine, made from polyunsaturated oil, is a good nutritional substitute for butter.

"About the only thing they have in common is that you can spread them on bread," says one of my biochemist friends. "Of course, you could do the same with shoe polish or library paste. Butter is far superior from the standpoint of food values."

A fact with tons of documentation is that when polyunsaturated oils are processed to make margarine, they become re-saturated. So much for margarine and polyunsaturated oils.

Let's look at the much maligned egg. Not many years ago he was a good egg. Actually, he still is, but you wouldn't know it if you relied on medical establishment information.

If any food can be called perfect, the egg can, inasmuch as it contains all the amino acids essential to our health. Over and above its protein richness, the egg boasts many vitamins: A, most of the B-complex (thiamin, riboflavin, pantothenic acid, pyridoxine, inositol, and biotin); D, E, and K; and minerals: calcium, chlorine, cobalt, copper, iodine, iron, magnesium, manganese, phosphorus, potassium, selenium, sodium, and zinc. Few foods are as digestible, contain as few calories, and cost as little per unit weight.

It is true that eggs are high in cholesterol. However, numerous research projects have shown that eating eggs has little or no effect on the blood cholesterol levels of most Americans. Only the 1 person in 500 with familial hypercholesterolemia or similar biochemical abnormality needs to minimize or eliminate eggs from the diet.

An experiment at the University of California School of Medicine in San Francisco involved feeding 1934 men and women up to fourteen eggs each week. Inasmuch as a large egg contains approximately 250 milligrams of cholesterol, researchers could find no statistically significant relationship between the quantity of eggs eaten and the blood serum cholesterol level.

Earlier, Dr. Roslyn Alfin-Slater and research associates at UCLA had been surprised to find that normal diets with increased egg intake did not elevate cholesterol levels.

Here is what she told a *Los Angeles Times* health reporter: "We, like everyone else, had been convinced that when you eat cholesterol, you get cholesterol. But when we stopped to think that all the studies in the past never tested the normal diet in relation to egg eating . . . we decided to see what happened to blood cholesterol levels on normal diets when egg intake was increased. Our finding surprised us. . . ."

Still another experiment, this one by Professor A.H. Ismail of Purdue University, confirmed the results of the UCLA researchers.

Does the once welcome egg deserve its bad press?

A resounding "No!" comes from researchers at Massachusetts Institute of Technology, who discovered that by eating two eggs daily, the individuals tested benefited from five grains of lecithin, a fat emulsifier, in the yolks. Within twenty-one days, this dietary regimen increased the plasma choline content of the brain by 500 percent, augmenting the synthesis of acetylcholine, the brain's key neurotransmitter. The bottom line of this study is that lecithin is helpful in restoring short-term memory loss.

In *Time* magazine Rockefeller University's Dr. Edward Ahrens, who has done cholesterol research for a generation, agreed that hypercholesterolemics should avoid high-cholesterol and high-fat foods, but not the rest of the population. Denying everybody eggs, dairy products, and meat when an infinitesimal fraction of the population has hypercholesterolemia is reducing one of the joys of living unnecessarily, he insists.

In the same issue of *Time* Purdue University cardiologist John Story scoffs at what he refers to as "cholesterolphobia," recommending that we not treat every resident of the land with diet, just as we don't give insulin to everyone for fear of their developing diabetes.

For a very good reason, many more authorities object to people restricting their intake of certain health-giving foods unnecessarily. When cholesterol from food is absorbed into the bloodstream, the self-regulatory system within us turns off the body's own production of this substance. Thus intake of cholesterol in the normal person does not necessarily raise the blood serum cholesterol level.

The American Heart Association would have us eat only two eggs a week. (I have never seen such an injunction in the Bible.) Another alternative, aside from eliminating them altogether, is using egg substitutes. Despite its name, this product doesn't beat eggs at all. It doesn't come close. Egg Beaters and similar man-made products made of egg whites, polyunsaturated oil, coloring, flavoring, and nutrients found in egg yolks contain no cholesterol and are supposed to be the same as eggs.

Are they?

You be the judge. Some years ago at the University of Illinois, baby rats were fed either egg substitutes or whole eggs. All the Egg Beaters eaters died within four weeks. The rats on whole eggs lived and remained in perfect health.

Rather than skip excellent, body-building foods such as milk, eggs, and butter—just a little of the last one—it is easier to cut fat intake in other ingredients of our diet from what could be a weight-gaining level of 40 to 45 percent of the total diet to 30 or 35 percent or less.

Here are some commonsense recommendations from Barbara Bassett, former editor and publisher of *Bestways*, a leading health and nutrition publication:

1. Never fail to remove skin from poultry prior to baking or roasting.
2. Slice off visible fat from all meat and poultry.
3. Always make soups and stews a day before use so that congealed fat can be skimmed off before reheating.
4. Eliminate cooking fats by browning foods in nonstick pans.
5. Replace calorie-loaded sour cream (for baked potatoes) with plain or low-fat yogurt. This kind of yogurt can also be blended with mayonnaise and used to finish sauces to reduce fat content and calories.
6. When in restaurants, control the amount of salad dressings and sauces used by ordering them on the side.
7. Instead of serving guests salads with dressings, offer them finger foods: carrot, celery, and green pepper sticks and radishes.
8. Use nonstick spray coating, preferably containing lecithin, rather than grease or butter on baking pans or casseroles.
9. Select low-fat, low-calorie mayonnaise and salad dressings in place of the usual kind.

10. Eat nuts in place of nut butters. Nut butters contain twice as many calories as the nuts from which they are made.

Lowering intake of dietary fat is a good idea for most individuals, even if they are not markedly overweight. Experiments by Dr. Jules Hirsch and associates at Rockefeller University disclose that eating a high-fat diet can cause a multiplication of fat cells, which are repositories for more fat.

What's so bad about that? The fact that once you develop a fat cell, you never lose it. The only thing you can do about it is lose enough weight so that the fat content of the cell is reduced. Dr. Hirsch's team, which includes Irving Faust and Rudolph Leibel, found that the fat cells of obese individuals are often two to two and a half times as large as those of people of average weight.

They also discovered that fat cells have two kinds of receptors on their surfaces: alpha and beta. Alpha receptors store fat and beta receptors break it down. Fat accumulates in certain places—belly or thighs—because there are more alpha than beta receptors there.

Several recent studies show that some of us may be predisposed by heredity to have more fat cells than others do, and more alpha than beta receptors. However, it is not a good idea to assume that you are genetically programmed to be overweight or obese. This will discourage you from even trying to win the losing game.

Remember, you can still win. Visualize fat cells as minute (actually microscopic), flexible, rubber bags, like mini-balloons. As they inflate, you inflate. With a combination of diet and exercise, you can reduce the size of those "cell balloons" and, with persistence, reduce your dimensions to a size you can live comfortably with in your clothing and in society.

A good start in the right direction involves gradually reducing the total amount of fat in your diet. I use the word "gradually" because an abrupt change can make it difficult to stick with your diet and you could slip off and be disheartened about getting back on again. You can easily live with a conservative reduction of fat and, if necessary, lower that by degrees until you achieve your weight goal.

CHAPTER EIGHT

OVERWEIGHT:
PERILS OF EXCESS
POUNDAGE

They are enclosed in their own fat . . . Psalms 17:10
(KJV)

*S*UPPOSEDLY, the ambitious man dies for fame, but the glutton dies for his belly. Neither reason seems praiseworthy, particularly the latter.

The pleasure of living to eat is usually followed by the pain of "dying" to lose weight.

At the start of this chapter is the Bible verse, "They are enclosed in their own fat." Believe me, "enclosed" is the right word, because excess fat is indeed a prison whose emotional punishments are self-dislike, low self-esteem, depression, and despair.

Obesity can also bring on a medical book full of physical disorders and even premature death. What really are the chances for survival of the fattest? Worse than those for the merely overweight and much worse than those for the lean.

Numerous studies reveal the glaring fact that obesity and even moderate overweight with a certain distribution of fat contribute to myriad ailments, minor to major, including heart and artery problems, high blood pressure, diabetes, and even cancer.

It is not my purpose to frighten you with gloom and doom prospects but to offer useful information that will motivate you to beat your weight problem.

Let's deal with first things first—cardiovascular conditions, inasmuch as they cause more hospitalizations and deaths, almost 500,000, each year in the United States than any other category of major illness.

Allen B. Nichols, M.D., and colleagues at the University of Michigan School of Medicine studied almost the entire population of Tecumseh, Michigan. They discovered that obesity and less extreme overweight raise the blood levels of cholesterol and triglycerides (which contribute to cardiovascular disorders) more than foods eaten.

Quite a few studies show that the cargo of excess fat carried around by the obese puts a strain on the heart that makes it work extra hard. Losing weight helps relieve the stress on the heart, which can only rest between beats.

Numerous studies disclose that hypertension (high blood pressure) commonly exists with obesity, putting a heavy burden on the heart, mainly on the left ventricle. Obesity and high blood pressure also invite congestive heart failure, coronary heart disease, and sudden death. Appreciable weight loss reduces blood pressure and cardiac output.

A study of 5500 male and female subjects aged 24 to 64 by the National Heart Foundation of Australia showed that obesity is definitely associated with blood pressure levels. Thirty percent of hypertension could be attributed to overweight. This study also revealed that 60 percent of the hypertension in men under age 45 was directly related to overweight. Even individuals who are just a bit overweight, along with the obese, can benefit in lower blood-pressure from losing excess poundage.

Obesity-caused high blood pressure is often passed on to the next generation. A Swedish study indicates that the sins of the father and mother are indeed visited upon the children.

A comparison of 121 hypertensives and 138 nonhypertensives highlighted the finding that children are more likely to develop high blood pressure when parents are both obese and hypertensive, than if they are just hypertensive. In considering excess poundage as a threat to health, we usually think in terms of fat distributed throughout the body. Now many studies disclose that heavy men and women with abdominal obesity are most likely to develop ischemic heart disease (medicalese for too little blood supply to the Big Pump).

A review of medical literature in the *Annals of Clinical Research* indicates that even those who have only limited abdominal obesity should not be complacent. Dieting and regular aerobic exercise can help get rid of this threatening condition.

Simple exercises can help you spot reduce:

1. Lying on your back, just raise your legs slowly, bottoms of your feet toward the ceiling, then let them down slowly. Start with five or ten times or whatever is your beginning capability. Then increase it by fives up to fifty.
2. Lying flat on your back, cross one straightened-out leg over the other, touching the floor on the opposite side. Then do this with the other leg. Start with ten for each leg or whatever you can do, increasing to twenty-five for each leg.
3. Accompany these exercises with thirty or more minutes of brisk walking, jogging, or bike riding every day.

Always get your doctor's approval if there's any doubt about your physical capability to do these exercises.

An excellent question I often get after my health lectures is, "How can I tell if my paunch is large enough to be hazardous to my health?"

Any oversize paunch could be hazardous, but the *Annals of Clinical Research* study cited above suggests using a tape measure. If the circumference of your waist is larger than that of your hips, better work to reduce it.

The risk factor of the big belly was suspected for some years by authorities in bariatrics, but it was unequivocally documented by a 13-year study of 722 fifty-four-year-old male residents of Gothenburg, Sweden. This study showed that the waist-to-hip circumference ratio is significant to the incidence of stroke and ischemic heart disease.

Here is the essence of the study in the researchers' words:

". . . In middle-aged men, the distribution of fat deposits may be a better predictor of cardiovascular disease and death than the degree of adiposity."

Aside from heart attacks, individuals with a fat belly also show increased risk of high blood pressure, as indicated by a study of 5506 test subjects aged 30 to 59, reported in the American Journal of Epidemiology (April, 1984).

Something that Dr. Rudolph Leibel, a long-time Rockefeller University researcher, told a conference of the American Heart Association about the hazards of body fat sounds similar to the three cardinal principles about the value of real estate: "location, location, location."

He said that the location of fat in the wrong place, the belly area, not only imposes a far greater risk of cardiovascular disease but also of many other ailments. Belly fat—the "spare tire," "the bay window," or the "Milwaukee Goiter"—is more detrimental to health than the total amount of fat a person is hauling around.

We women might complain about the tendency of body fat to home in on our hips, thighs, and behinds, but at least it doesn't go to the waist, as with men. The waist is the danger zone, and, according to Leibel, it is one of the reasons women live longer than men. He says that some men who are not particularly fat but have a "beer gut" are "walking time bombs."

Research by Leibel and his associates shows that an enlarged belly can triple the risk of cardiovascular disease and sharply increase the threat of stroke and diabetes.

Why is fat around the mid-section so much more damaging than in other parts of the anatomy?

Referring to various studies, Leibel states that fatty tissue in the stomach floods the liver with fatty acids. This overflow interferes with the liver's ability to control blood levels of insulin. The consequence of this could be diabetes and greater risk of cardiovascular disease, because then blood pressure becomes elevated and the body holds more sodium.

Leibel feels it is of critical importance to burn off excess fat around the mid-section. So, build in a measure of safety as you eliminate the middle man, or woman.

Fat banks in the buttocks, hips, and thighs in no way affect the liver, says Leibel, who claims that women tend to become pear-shaped because of their potential for becoming mothers. He states that fat cells are stockpiles of energy and that 80,000 calories of warehoused fat are necessary for women to become pregnant. Abdominal fat can interfere with menstrual cycles by limiting production of insulin, so women were created in such a way that fat could be stored elsewhere—in the buttocks, hips, and thighs.

Several scientists including Leibel have discovered that women have more fat cells in these body areas than men because they have two times as much lipoprotein lipase, an enzyme that attracts fat cells like a magnet attracts iron filings.

Men have more alpha receptors on their bellies. These block fat from leaving the cells. However, a weight reduction regimen such as the Diet Bible diet, outlined in chapter 25, can bring about weight loss in all parts of the body.

A few paragraphs ago mention was made that abdominal fat can contribute to diabetes, a blood sugar disorder that plagues some 11 million Americans. Almost constantly elevated blood sugar levels indicates a breakdown of the body's energy use system. A simple sugar, glucose, is the high-octane fuel that gives us energy and heat. Circulating blood transports sugar to our trillions of body cells, but something more than delivery is needed.

To pass through the cell walls, glucose needs to become attached to biochemical ushers: tiny molecules of the pancreatic hormone insulin. When there's an insulin shortage, as in diabetes, sugar accumulates and wanders helplessly in the blood. It finally enters the kidneys to be excreted in the urine.

Obesity is a physiological form of stress that invites diabetes by means of the spillage of fatty acids from the abdominal areas into the liver, as described by Leibel. This spillage can also occur from the blood in times of emotional or physical stress, shutting off the release of insulin.

Dr. W. John Butterfield, professor of medicine at Guys Hospital in London and a respected authority on diabetes, observes a remarkable similarity between the manner in which the body handles sugar in diabetes and in conditions of obesity and slightly lesser overweight.

Butterfield experimented to test comparative glucose uptake in three types of persons: those with juvenile diabetes, those with maturity onset diabetes (the most common kind), and normal controls of varying weights.

Juvenile diabetics showed no ability to absorb sugar into their cells. Older diabetics and obese normal test subjects were similar in their flawed ability to take up glucose. Lean individuals ab- sorbed more sugar than the plump ones.

In noting that obese test subjects handled—really, mis- handled—glucose nearly as diabetics do, Butterfield concludes that as obesity continues or increases, less insulin can reach in- sulin-responsive muscles. Therefore, increasingly less glucose is taken up, putting pressure on the pancreas gland to form more insulin.

As obesity increases and the number of cells to be serviced multiplies, the pancreas can't supply enough insulin to meet de- mand. Result? Constantly elevated blood sugar.

Dr. Butterfield observes that obese individuals are diabetes- prone because body fat competes with lean tissue such as muscle for the available insulin, and the fat wins. Then glucose is changed into fat.

As with cardiovascular conditions, one study reveals that diabetes can result from fat located in certain specific body loca- tions. Prominent fat in the upper body can more readily move individuals over the line into diabetes than can generally distrib- uted fat.

A fascinating revelation about diet, obesity, and diabetes is given by Associate Professor Somasundaram Addanki, of the Ohio State University College of Medicine. He is a diabetic who married a diabetic.

Addanki, a biochemist, and his wife did not develop diabetes until they left their native India and began eating "the typical high-fat, high sugar, and low fiber diet consumed in western countries," as he writes in the journal *Preventive Medicine*. He explains how this poor diet turns healthy individuals into dia- betics.

Fatty, low-fiber, sugary foods encourage certain intestinal bacteria to produce overabundant estrogen, one of the female hormones. Further, an enzyme in body fat joins up with testos- terone, the male hormone, to produce more estrogen, which makes the cells of skeletal muscles insensitive to the action of insulin. This is where the merely overweight and the obese come in.

With additional weight gain, additional insulin is needed. Continued stress on the pancreas gland synthesizes a greater amount of insulin, and this gland becomes exhausted, bringing on extra-high blood sugar and the medical disorder called diabetes.

Inasmuch as testosterone is central to male sexual urge and potency, the Addanki "excess estrogen" theory reveals why obese adult males often become impotent and obese women often develop a greater sexual drive. Explaining his theory in a United Press International story, Addanki reveals that he had experienced "six years of diabetic impotency," prior to a dietary change that helped him control his disease.

Addanki's advice to all fat people who want to prevent diabetes is simple and helpful: Avoid eating sugar, white flour, and fatty foods.

Over and above obesity as a Trojan Horse factor in undermining health is the duration of this abnormal condition. How long unwelcome fat stays determines the extent of the physical damage. One study discloses that long-time obesity causes the heart's left ventrical wall to thicken and changes the heart's dimension, its stroke volume, and output.

In one study thirty-five obese subjects of the same approximate weight and fat cell size were divided into two groups: those who had been obese for less than fifteen years and those who had been so for more than fifteen years. The two groups were compared with a normal-weight control group.

In this comparison the two groups of obese patients manifested enlargement of the heart's ventricles and abnormalities of heart performance. Predictably, the group who had been obese for a longer period had markedly thicker heart ventricle walls and greater ventricular dimension. This proved to researchers that the longer obesity persists, the more harm is done.

An insight into how well the body recovers from the damage of obesity was provided in a related study, in which substantial weight loss helped to reverse left ventricle dysfunction to some extent.

Another cardiovascular condition that usually responds to weight reduction by lower food intake and more exercise is high blood pressure. Elevated blood pressure often starts declining well before weight loss reduces a person to so-called normal size.

Several studies accent the fact that blood pressure can often be lowered significantly not only by the obese but also by individuals who are moderately to slightly overweight. An experiment underscores this point. Fifty-six young, overweight test subjects with a diastolic blood pressure of 90 to 109—that's the resting phase of the heart—were divided into two groups. One group tried to control hypertension by reducing weight; the other group took an anti-hypertensive drug, metoprolol. A control group took placebos.

Twenty-one weeks later, the weight losers had dropped an average of sixteen pounds, and their systolic pressure had fallen thirteen points—significant compared with the placebo group's seven-point drop, but not much improved over the metoprolol takers' ten-point drop.

Yet the bottom line for the diastolic pressure showed a distinct advantage for the weight losers: a ten-point decline. This compares with six points for the metoprolol takers and just three for the placebo group.

The improvement in blood fats made the weight losers look even better. Their blood cholesterol level decreased, and so did their ratio of total cholesterol to high-density lipoproteins (HDL, the beneficial cholesterol).

Patients on metoprolol had no such beneficial results: Their blood cholesterol increased and their HDL level dropped.

Another experiment, involving forty obese women, resulted in weight loss again elevating HDL in comparison with LDL, which means improved insurance against cardiovascular disorders.

Combining diet and exercise proved even more effective in raising HDL in comparison with LDL, as an experiment with twenty-one obese sedentary males showed.

Obesity seems to encourage all sorts of disorders; cancer, diabetes (already covered), gallstones, and respiratory ailments are among the most important categories.

An American Cancer Society study over a twelve-year period led to the discovery that obesity increases the risk of a wide range of cancers in both sexes: breast, colon, gallbladder, kidney, stomach, and uterus. Frightening facts about the hazards of overweight emerged from this study. Overweight women are at a far greater risk than men to develop cancer. In comparing the proneness of 40-percent-overweight women and men, the ACS researchers discovered the women to be at 55 percent greater risk than their normal-weight counterparts, while the men were 33 percent more cancer-prone than normal-weights.

Still another study informed researchers that though obesity doesn't seem to cause breast cancer, it does apparently encourage the spread of existing cancer.

Not generally known is the fact that obesity contributes to a type of malignancy exclusive to males: cancer of the prostate. In a twenty-year study by Seventh Day Adventists of 6763 white males, it was discovered that overweight males develop a much higher amount of prostate cancers than their normal-weight counterparts.

There is hardly an area of the body or a physiological activity that is not negatively influenced by obesity.

Even female sex organs and pregnancy are complicated by obesity, as discovered by researchers who made a gigantic search of controlled studies covering 10,440 cases over twenty-two years. The best documented obesity-complicated problems in pregnancy were: preeclampsia, diabetes mellitus, varicose veins, and the requirement for caesarean section. One aspect of this study surprised even the researchers, however: that birthweight of infants from obese mothers, although significantly higher than that of infants from normal-weight mothers, caused no increase in labor complications.

Still another medical disorder promoted by obesity is gallbladder trouble in both sexes. Massively obese patients do not achieve good results with the conventional treatment, cheno-deoxycholic acid.

One particular physical complication of obesity rarely escapes the patient's attention: difficulty in breathing caused by fat-restricting chest expansion and inbreathing, as reported in the medical journal *Respiration*. Unless the patient loses appreciable weight, this condition becomes worse with time because the pressure of fat limits lung capacity, flow of air, and even the out-breathing of carbon dioxide.

Yet, restricted respiration does not complete the list of key medical complications caused by obesity, as revealed by observation and test of twelve massively obese patients ranging from 312 to 500 pounds. Seven patients were diagnosed as having hypertension; four had sleep apnea (erratic breathing); two had diabetes mellitus, and one had coronary artery disease. Five patients died suddenly—two from right-sided congestive heart failure, one from acute myocardial infarction, one from aortic dissection, one from intracerebral hemorrhage, one from drug overdose, and one from an ileal bypass.

The heart seems to take the worst stress from obesity; it has to force five quarts of blood through hundreds of pounds of flesh and fat. And does the stress show? Every one of the patients in the study manifested heart abnormality: increased heart weight, dilation of the left ventricular heart cavity in eleven test subjects, and the same condition in the right ventricular cavity in twelve.

One of the corrective measures some obese and even moderate heavyweights pursue is fasting, the subject of the next chapter.

HOW NOT TO EAT YOURSELF TO DEATH

. . . The drunkard and glutton shall come to poverty
. . . Proverbs 23:21 (KJV)

*T*HE only reason two of the most famous gluttons in history didn't eat themselves out of house and home is that they lived in palaces. It's a good arrangement, but it's hard to come by these days. You could scan the classified ads for years and not find many openings for emperors.

No records exist that show whether or not the appetites of two Roman emperors, Vitellius and Maximin, made it necessary to raise taxes, but we know they brought on inflation—not only to their waistlines but also to their fat heads.

Vitellius was the greatest glutton to eat his way into history. He is supposed to have swilled up 1000 oysters a day for eight months, eating from a huge $100,000 silver platter called the Shield of Minerva. Within this eight-month period, he alone ate $90,000 worth of gourmet foods: flamingo tongues, livers of parrot fish, peacock brains, and lamprey milk.

The *New Columbia Encyclopedia* says that his rule was distinguished by "extravagance, debauchery and general incompetence." A rival faction defeated him militarily and murdered him —a drastic way of killing his appetite.

Maximin, too, was quite a physical specimen: eight feet tall—what an NBA center he would have made!—and, eventually, with a matching circumference. A barbarian with incredible

77

physical prowess, he worked his way up to emperor. One historical account says he could pull a heavily loaded sledge and tear up small trees. In a day he drank seven gallons of wine and ate up to forty pounds of meat, among other tidbits.

He lasted three years as emperor and then was killed by his soldiers during a siege. It is said that the end of his wine and food budget permitted the financing of another military campaign. (That may not be history, but it makes good reading.)

Some other world-famous gluttons—England's famous diarist Samuel Pepys and Queen Elizabeth I, France's King Charles V, and, America's William Jennings Bryan, the great orator and presidential also-ran—subsisted on austerity diets compared with the Roman Emperors.

Most of these individuals who lived to eat didn't live to eat for long. Their Epicurean philosophy, "Eat, drink and be merry, for tomorrow we die," turned out to be a self-fulfilling prophecy.

Noted nineteenth-century physician Oliver Wendell Holmes supposedly said that "Surfeiting (overfeeding) has destroyed more lives than starving." That's hard to prove statistically, Oliver, but it seems true.

What actually happens to the human anatomy when the stomach is overwhelmed with far more food than it can readily process? More than you know.

Not enough digestive enzymes can by synthesized for the landslide of food. Therefore, some of the food remains undigested, so putrefactive bacteria that cause gas multiply. Overindulgers eat overfast and swallow air, adding to stomach and intestinal distension.

Perhaps the best alternative to copious amounts of food at one or two sittings is numerous small meals. Dr. Richard Passwater, a prominent biochemist and author of the best-selling *Supernutrition*, permitted laboratory animals to eat as frequently as they wished, and they flourished. On one or two meals of the same caloric value as that of the total of smaller feedings, they gained weight.

Passwater suggests our eating five or six small meals daily to prevent overloading and overworking our complex digestion and transport system. Heavy intakes of food put great strain on reserves of various organs, including the heart, he states.

Intakes of food that dwarf capacity for digestion and absorption cause another complication. Just imagine that your trillions of cells are micro-carburetors; they can only process a finite amount of fuel at one time. After the cells' needs have been satisfied, the extra glucose continues circulating.

However, because so much sugar is making the rounds in the bloodstream, more insulin must be secreted by the pancreas, overtaxing this organ. Insulin is the biochemical escort that ensures that blood glucose can enter the cells. Now it must muscle all that excess glucose into the cells until they can no longer burn enough of it.

So what happens? The excess glucose is translated into fat. As mini-droplets of fat accumulate, the cells balloon out to capacity. Overstuffing with food for month after month and year after year can even cause new fat cells to develop in the grossly obese. Old and new cells eventually become overfilled and will accept just the amount of blood glucose they need to burn and energize themselves. Despite this, stress is still exerted on the pancreas to secrete more insulin and force more glucose into the cells.

A medical term describes this state: end-organ resistance to insulin. It is seen in connective tissue and heart and skeletal muscles of the obese and diabetics. Inordinate pressure is put on the pancreas at this point. As end-organ resistance becomes more stubborn—characteristic in obese and diabetic individuals—secretion of insulin multiplies. Multiplies is the right word. Discharge of insulin per given amount of glucose, even in nondiabetic obese or otherwise heavyweight patients, becomes two to four times greater than in nonobese and nondiabetic patients. It is easy to see how the pancreas can become exhausted.

Now the vicious circle becomes even more vicious. Giant pendulum swings from overabundant blood sugar to too little cause nonstop hunger, which creates an insatiable urge to overeat. The overstuffed fat cells can hold no more fat, and insulin production steps up until the exhausted pancreas refuses to work anymore. Since there's not much of a market for used pancreases, it pays to be kind to the only one you've got.

Overeating and obesity can also contribute to liver malfunction. Biopsies in seriously overweight patients showed liver damage in every case; all individuals manifested subnormal liver function. Such injury to the liver, a biochemical enzyme factory, limits its ability to synthesize enough energy-producing enzymes. Thus fuel cannot be burned up fast enough and, as a result, fat accumulates.

One of the major contributors to liver damage is a diet high in refined carbohydrates. A study of 102 patients living mainly on junk food virtually devoid of protein showed, by means of weekly needle biopsies, that with an augmented diet—rich in protein and supplemented by choline, methionine, and vitamin B-12—the patients regained full liver function in six weeks. In instances in which the food supplement lecithin was used as the source of choline, recovery was even faster. The researchers conjecture that intestinal bacteria in some individuals destroy the vitamin choline.

An amazing organ, the liver can regenerate itself if given half a nutritional break. A rat whose liver was two-thirds surgically removed was given a diet rich in proteins, the vitamin B-complex, (with emphasis on choline), and vitamins C and E. It experienced a total liver regrowth in three weeks.

Another biochemical disaster can occur to the liver: an inability to synthesize enzymes needed to deactivate insulin, due to a diet low in protein, vitamin B-2, and/or pantothenic acid. Superfluous insulin coursing through the vascular system encourages fat to form rapidly and makes blood sugar plummet.

You may know this condition without being introduced: hypoglycemia. A hypoglycemic person adds weight quickly and has trouble losing it, mainly because of a constant and voracious appetite. As with liver damage, low blood sugar can be corrected without much difficulty by minimizing or eliminating refined carbohydrates (including alcohol), skipping caffeine, which causes release of liver-stored sugar, not smoking, adding complex carbohydrates and more protein to the diet, and eating five to six small meals daily rather than three big or moderate ones.

Rather than eat in this manner, ancient Roman royalty and nobility seemed to live for their banquets—formal nonstop binges—in which they gorged and then voluntarily or involuntarily vomited their food and came back for more. As a matter of fact, forced throwing-up in the manner of today's victims of bulimia was standard practice of upper classes in ancient Rome, where, for this very purpose, a regurgitorium was installed in their villas.

Psychophysical disorders such as anorexia nervosa and bulimia are not uncommon today. Anorexia, a condition of depressed appetite mainly in adolescent girls, involves a phobia of gaining weight and seems to drive victims to starve themselves to the point of facial emaciation and body distortion such as "razor blade hips," as characterized by a friend.

Anorexics visualize themselves as much heavier than they actually are and therefore try to conform to an artificial or imaginary physical standard. Some authorities claim that anorexia nervosa is caused or encouraged by a deficiency of zinc in the diet, and studies indicate that this claim may actually be valid.

Thirty hospitalized anorexics who found foods to be tasteless or at least uninviting were thought to be zinc-deficient and given 30 milligrams of zinc a day. Almost immediately, foods began to taste better and the patients' appetites picked up. Researchers couldn't draw a definite conclusion as whether or not zinc deficiency is an actual cause of this condition or whether it is merely associated with anorexia's symptoms. Whatever the answer, it worked in thirty out of thirty cases.

Anorexia nervosa and bulimia are sometimes experienced by the same person. It is difficult to trace their relationship to root causes. Bulimia, whose meaning is "ox hunger," or a voracious appetite, is characterized by binge eating—the sudden downing of prodigious amounts of food in a brief period.

These binges don't usually cause overweight or obesity because the bulimic induces vomiting as soon as possible after eating. Biochemist Jeffrey Bland estimates that there are approximately four bulimics to one anorexic.

Almost half of those with anorexia nervosa experience bulimic binges, some 43 percent of those having two or three binges a week. What emotional pressures induce the bulimic's inordinate lust for food? Over and above honest hunger are boredom, emptiness of life, frustration, and other stressors.

A binge followed by an emptying of the stomach rids the patient of the immediate pressure, but there is always the hovering specter of fear that she will not be able to stop eating. Also, powerful digestive juices that gush out with the food often burn and irritate the throat and contribute to erosion of tooth enamel and consequent decay.

Some authorities believe that bulimia is caused by a specific menstrual disorder: amenorrhea, abnormal absence of menstruation caused by hormonal imbalance. Many cases of amenorrhea and other menstrual disorders have been traced to hypothyroidism, or low thyroid function. Stephen Langer, M.D., a preventive medicine specialist of Berkeley, California, has had success treating several bulimia cases as symptomatic of low thyroid function, and prescribing Armour natural desiccated thyroid.

Because there are certain common threads in bulimia and anorexia nervosa, Dr. Bland feels that zinc supplementation might also be useful in bulimia, accompanied by a high-potency vitamin B-complex regimen and psychological counseling.

High-profile characteristics of the bulimic and the anorexic are almost identical: highly intelligent, hard-charging, and goal-oriented, with standards so high they are frequently "the unreachable star." Often these personalities keep raising their goals to make them virtually impossible for a human being to reach.

Consequently, bulimics and anorexics seek to compensate for frustration by binge eating associated with fear of a real or imagined physical imperfection, focalized on weight. Bland finds these same characteristics in male compulsive runners, indicative of the fact that these two types of compulsives show an abnormal fear of overweight.

James Braly, M.D., a prominent Encino, California allergist and director of Optimum Health Labs there, maintains that much gluttony is caused by an addiction some individuals have to certain foods, on which they binge. Braly believes that the major and most common reason for overeating in the Western world is the "Siamese twin" disorder: food allergy/food addiction.

Encouraging food allergy/food addiction is the fact that we eat a severely limited number of foods and eat them too often. With hundreds of different foods available, Americans get some 80 percent of their calories from just eleven, which are on the list of most commonly allergenic foods in the book, *Dr. Braly's Optimum Health Program.* Presented alphabetically these foods are: beef, cheese, chocolate, citrus fruit (orange), coffee, corn, eggs, malt, milk, peanuts, pork, potato (white), rye, spices (various), soybeans, tomato, and whole wheat. Eating the same foods again and again invites allergy.

Beyond the sensitivities or allergies these foods can cause for many of us is a condition Dr. Braly calls "leaky gut" syndrome. With some 3000 chemical substances added to our foods and another 10,000 chemical contaminants that enter our food or us unintentionally, we develop a permeable intestinal lining that allows partially digested food particles to filter through into our bloodstream. Foods eaten with coffee or an alcoholic beverage slip through the intestinal lining more readily.

Unlike totally digested foods, these large molecules appear to the immune system to be threatening enemy invaders, or allergens. They trigger an antibody response, and the immune system works to conquer them and get them out of the blood.

Being susceptible to allergy is mainly a matter of leakiness of the gut—permitting substances that don't belong there into the bloodstream. Braly says that leaky gut syndrome related to even moderate alcohol drinking offers an explanation of the basics of allergy/addiction to both foods and alcohol.

Superimposed upon all this is the naked fact that we eat too much food—something like 500 to 1000 calories above our actual requirements for maintaining good health. This overwhelming volume suppresses the immune system, as demonstrated by numerous, well-structured animal experiments that have shown that reducing the caloric intake of animals—while maintaining them above the level of malnourishment—has led to their living almost twice as long as the control group and with a lower incidence of cancer and other degenerative disorders associated with aging.

So many of us become philosophical or martyrs about weight gain, fatigue, aches and pain, swelling under the eyes, sneezes and wheezes, and irritability and depression for no reason that we can put our finger on. We may never suspect that it is a food allergy and related malnourishment that underlies the problem. Suddenly we're struck by a lightning bolt of serious illness and the immune system, overstressed by battling against allergy, has too little reserves to overcome the disease and protect us.

The body adapts in the best way it knows to repeated food and environmental allergens. It races to the battle front with stress chemicals and other biochemical defenders and mediators to cushion the suffering caused by the allergic foods. The combination of these chemicals and hormones temporarily relieves the discomfort or pain and brings a high mood.

A low follows. Subconsciously we crave the allergenic food to loft us back to the high. The return of lows and then the consumption of allergenic foods to give us another lift makes us addicts. Strangely, the addictive foods really don't make us feel great. They just relieve us from feeling miserable.

The allergy/addiction syndrome is at the root of most food allergies. How to get rid of the allergy? Break the addiction, mainly by learning our food allergens and then studiously eliminating them.

It is hard to say whether it was food allergy that developed binge eating in one of the fattest men ever to live in the United States: Happy Humphrey, of Augusta, Georgia, who depressed the scales with 802 pounds.

Even as a baby he was an oversized 18 pounds. A bit later, his parents diapered him with a bedsheet. His appetite was prodigious from the start. By the time he was 12 years old, he weighed around 300 pounds.

Happy could never remember any period of his life when he wasn't fat. He admits that eating to him was like drinking to an alcoholic. He just couldn't stop. Once he was old enough to be on his own, he could hardly make enough money to feed himself let alone provide for normal expenses of living. Happy easily ate a fourteen-pound turkey with all the trimmings at a sitting. And he often consumed fifteen chickens at a time.

Happy knew he had to reduce when, during a wrestling match, he suffered a heart attack. Under doctor's orders, he was told to lose weight, and by sheer will and grit he was able to melt down from 802 to 644. Then it became hard to lose, and Happy became a volunteer patient at the Medical College of Georgia Clinical Investigation Unit.

Dr. Wayne Greenberg put Happy Humphrey in the hospital and over the months, under controlled conditions, supervised his losing down to a slender 227 pounds. Humphrey was never fed less than 1000 calories daily and was put on special diets in fifty-six day cycles.

During the first twenty-eight-day part of the cycle, he was given three meals a day and a bedtime snack, with the same food served every day. It is a wonder that these food repetitions didn't cause an allergic reaction in Humphrey and stop his weight loss.

In the next twenty-eight days, he ate the same foods but took in all his calories from one meal. One-third of the time he ate mainly fat foods. One-third of the time he ate mainly carbohydrates. In the last third he ate mainly protein. The high-protein diet brought the most rapid weight loss. On this diet Humphrey ate ground beef twice daily.

Humphrey was elated with being able to lose so much poundage. Many factors pleased him. For the first time since he could remember, he could cross his legs. Other never-before-possible things he could do were hunt, fish, and swim. For the first time in fifteen years, he could sleep lying down. Before, he was so big that he had to sleep at a 45-degree angle. His biggest boost, however, was in being able to wear store-bought clothes.

The story of Happy Humphrey, whose real name is William J. Cobb, shows that the impossible—losing almost 600 pounds—is possible, even for someone whose life was one binge of gluttonous eating.

No one said it was easy—particularly not Happy Humphrey—but it is possible. Happy Humphrey knows. He did it.

CHAPTER TEN

TO FAST OR NOT TO FAST . . .

I humbled my soul with fasting, and my prayer returned to my bosom . . . Psalms 35:13 (KJV)

*O*NE widespread misconception prevents many overweight and obese individuals from trying the total fast.

"Why go on it?" ask many who attend my lectures, "When it's over, you just defeat the purpose by eating that much more."

'Tain't necessarily so!

After a lengthy, total fast most individuals can handle only a small amount of food, as is demonstrated when long-term, semi-starved prisoners of war are released. I heard about a man who had been on a thirty-five-day fasting diet, ate a small orange, and was unable to keep it down.

It is true, however, that after two or three years, 50 percent of the total fasters regain all the poundage they lost through fasting, as one study shows. Fewer than 10 percent were able to retain their lower weight after nine years.

Because this less than 10 percent fascinates me, I have interviewed quite a few individuals who were able to keep their new slender figure for five or ten years after total fasting. What was the strength they gained from fasting that enabled them to do it?

Part of that strength is secular; The other part is spiritual. Relative to secular strength, something profoundly moving happens to the obese during a lengthy fast: a feeling of control and power over the fat. This sense of power carries over for years. If they could desist from food completely for thirty-five days, they can live with limited caloric intake forever. They gain further reinforcement—a stainless steel determination—from the benefits of a new public and private image: enhanced social and career opportunities, elevated self-esteem, and greater good health and well-being.

The spiritual benefits come from the euphoria that many fasters experience—a freedom from the heavy anchor of the body, a closeness to God. It is like the feeling expressed in the Bible verse at the start of this chapter: "I humbled my soul with fasting, and my prayer returned to mine bosom." This deliverance from captivity of the body releases prayer, which in turn enlists divine help for remaining less heavy.

The previous chapter mentioned the major physical disorders to which the obese, other heavyweights, and those with a paunch are often prone. One of my biochemist friends estimates that gross overweight can cause or intensify more than sixty physical ailments, plus a swarm of nagging and persistent emotional problems.

Is it hard to adhere to a fast?

Indeed! However, no total fast should be attempted outside of a hospital with doctors always on hand. Hospital personnel offer emotional support and discipline. Here's a frank statement from a formerly obese person who suffered through fasting:

"The first days—as a matter of fact, the first week—is agony. All I could think about was food. I almost hallucinated food, like a parched-throated, lost-in-the-desert person experiences the illusion of an oasis. I would hate to go through it again. And this now helps to make me monitor my appetite and stay at a reasonable weight."

What about after the first week?

"There's no craving for food. It was a wonderful release after a lifetime of being food-compelled—an incredible feeling of power, self-satisfaction, and new self-esteem."

Don't let these glowing words mislead you. Total fasting, unlike the one-day-a-week juice fasting practiced by many Christians, puts the human body through inhuman stress.

My friend Luke Bucci, chief biochemist of Biotics, Inc., tells me:

"In fasting, despite all this business you hear about blood being cleansed, vitamins and minerals are depleted—nutrients necessary to cope with the death of cells which cannot be replaced without these required nutrients.

"The liver is under inordinate strain, because it has to translate fat into energy. The kidneys, too, are under dire stress because they must handle and excrete overwhelming amounts of biochemical byproducts of the breakdown of fat and protein."

Further, when fat is burned a residue like ash from a fire remains—ketones—giving rise to a condition called ketosis, which helps to elevate blood uric acid, which can lead into gout. It is believed by some authorities that ketosis may be the condition that kills appetite in fasters.

Common to fasting is bad breath, which in some instances would wither a redwood tree. However, this condition is the least of a laundry list of physical problems: depressed metabolic rate, and consequent slowing of heart rate with sluggish delivery of oxygen-carrying blood, and diminished muscle strength and coordination.

D.R. Young, M.D., a research scientist with the National Aeronautics and Space Administration, has found that in starvation—total fasting is voluntary starvation—the greater amount of fat supporting the intestines is lost, compared with that in tissues under the skin—at a ratio of 50 to 30 percent.

According to Dr. Young, fasting burns up not only fat and body protein but also protein from organs whose function is critical to our very existence: the heart, kidneys, and liver. Liver and kidney damage is not uncommon.

Other undermining conditions often resulting are hypotension (low blood pressure), accompanying light-headedness or dizziness, heart arrhythmia, spasms of the hands, headaches, nausea, hair loss, dry mouth, sleeplessness, loss of sex drive, and mild to extreme depression. Dr. Young discovered that a 300-pound person who has lost half his weight by means of incomplete or total starvation may be mired so deep in depression that he could be close to attempting suicide.

So far we have dealt with specific physical ailments that can develop from fasting, but what biochemical mechanisms does fasting bring on?

First, there's a drain on the glucose supply, the major fuel for the brain. In the initial stages of fasting, the body sends an SOS to the liver for its glycogen reserves, which, according to need, are converted to blood sugar. Without food fuels to produce more glucose, the body next eats into its protein supply, starting with the muscles. Programmed for survival, the body starts translating fat into glucose before the protein supply is near depletion.

Next in the survival process, the brain, in its hunger, desperately signals the body to "do something" about its food supply, and the body responds in a last ditch operation, converting about all that's left—ketones, the by-product of burning of fat for fuel.

Fasting consumes a great deal of water, which is why fasters must take in inordinate amounts of fluid. It also depletes minerals—sodium, potassium, calcium, magnesium, and phosphate. Potassium loss contributes to low blood pressure.

One of the most devastating stressors in fasting is exhaustion of the adrenal glands—a characteristic of which is low blood sugar—which contributes to a ravenous appetite and a craving for sweets.

With these tremendous strains on body and mind, it is obvious that fasting is not for everybody. No one should go into it if physically or emotionally ill. Fasting is for the hardy blessed with stamina.

Garfield G. Duncan, M.D., of Pennsylvania Hospital in Philadelphia, is a recognized authority on fasting and starvation. He warns that the following individuals should not attempt fasting: pregnant women and patients with infections, liver problems, peptic ulcers, and diabetes.

Traditional medicine rarely cautions the public about one of the greatest dangers of fasting. Even worse, it does not usually take measures to cope with the problem in patients hospitalized for total fasting.

Gary Gordon, M.D., founder of the American College of Advancement in Medicine, and head of the Preventive Medicine Clinic of Sacramento, has an effective way of coping with a frightening complication of modern-day fasting, which some call "flirting with suicide."

"Fasting is particularly stressful on the body because toxins are stored in the fat," says Dr. Gordon. "We could be said to be swimming in a sea of toxins. Everyone tests positive for PCB, DDT, and the many other chlorinated pesticides used commonly in our homes, gardens and food supply. This is true even of polar bears in the Arctic."

"Burning fat in the fasting process means you are releasing toxins into the bloodstream. The body must be protected from the toxic effects of these harmful chemicals," he states.

Dr. Gordon requires his patients to fast on vegetable juices for the first three days, with concentrated supplementary nutrients: the most strategic anti-oxidants, vitamins C, A, and E. Also, the body must be constantly cleansed internally with a fiber such as psyllium seed. Enemas or colonics done by a colon therapist keep toxins moving through the bowel so that they can't be absorbed. It is important to keep water going in at the rate of six to eight glasses daily for cleansing.

Dr. Gordon adds that some form of exercise is a must, especially the kind that makes you sweat. "Sweat has its own virtue for ridding the body of impurities and toxins. The largest organ for both absorption and elimination is the skin. It is important to perform some daily aerobic exercise that causes sweating. If that is impossible, the sauna or steam bath can bring on sweating."

After the third day, Dr. Gordon starts his fasters on amino acids to compensate for loss of lean muscle mass—six tablets a day of free-form amino acids, plus two fifty-mg vitamin B-6 tablets, important to transporting the amino acids.

Is the early agony of fasting worthwhile so far as losing specific amounts of weight are concerned? What do various research studies show?

Yes, indeed!

One study of 207 patients hospitalized to realize significant weight loss through continuous fasting demonstrated that 79 of them were successful in melting down to within 30 percent of their ideal weight. Most participants in this research project were able to maintain the amount of their weight reduction for at least a year and a half, no matter how much they lost. Two to three years later, one-half of these patients had returned to their original level of obesity.

I have talked to many individuals who managed dramatic and sizeable weight reduction through fasting and then gradually fell back into their former condition. Being free of fat had made them ecstatic. Now that they were again enslaved, they looked back wistfully at the past.

Dr. Gordon checked on more than one hundred patients who had lost weight by total fasting and discovered that 60 percent of them either continued to lose or maintained their new weight level. However, 40 percent gained everything back and more.

The experience of Ernst J. Drenick, M.D., with fasting patients at Wadsworth Veterans Administration Hospital in Los Angeles and at UCLA has shown that fasters can shed a pound a day and that the most obese show the greatest losses fastest. The amount of loss is the least in the leanest test subjects.

Dr. Drenick reports that women melt off weight more slowly than men, also that poundage disappears more quickly in the initial days of fasting and then levels off. One of his patients, a 540-pounder, dropped 71 pounds in the first month and 40 pounds the next. On a total fast, he states, individuals who weigh in at 230 pounds can realistically expect a loss of 35 pounds in a month.

Fasting makes taking it off easy, but a return to the usual eating habits makes putting it on easy as well. The regaining process is slow and subtle, but one morning you wake up and you're back where you started. This is the essence of findings by University of Dusseldorf researchers, who put forty-five heavyweights on a total fast for twelve days. (They did administer vitamin supplements, however.)

On an average, the test subjects lost twenty-eight pounds. Not one of the patients returned regularly to the clinic for a follow-up program. Of the forty-two patients who could be reached for a post-experiment interview, nine had regained all of their lost weight or more. Nineteen others had regained the biggest portion of their previous loss. Only fourteen had managed to keep their weight off or lose even more. Critics of this study state that the twelve-day fast was not long enough to break deeply entrenched dietary habits and consequently was a limited success.

The Dusseldorf researchers felt that their results were not quite on a par with those of Boston's George Blackburn, M.D., with his 300-calorie diet—actually, a modified fast. Dr. Black-

burn's patients lost dramatically, but 96 out of 105 patients regained all of their lost weight within two years.

Let's sum up the case for and against total fasting and pull
up the zipper on this chapter.

In Favor

1. The eating pattern contributory to excessive weight is broken by fasting, assuming that the period of fasting is the
   traditional thirty to sixty days.
2. A dramatic degree of weight loss that is actually visible
   and able to be sensed in other ways raises the patient's
   morale and helps her to see that permanent weight reduction is possible.
3. A new confidence, higher self-esteem, and a feeling of
   accomplishment comes to the long-time obese person
   through fasting.
4. New acceptability socially and in employment reinforces
   for the heavy person the belief that fasting has been worthwhile and establishes a base for more moderate eating in
   the future.
5. The faster achieves improved health and lowers susceptibility to obesity-induced or, -worsened diseases. In instances in which the paunch is seriously reduced, chances
   of developing cardiovascular disorders or diabetes are
   greatly lessened.

Against

1. Low blood pressure can be developed temporarily, causing dizziness and even fainting.
2. Kidney and liver damage can be sustained. Inasmuch as
   the liver can be regenerated, damage to it can usually be
   overcome. Kidney damage may not be completely re-
   versible. (However, I have just learned that the Preventive
   Medical Clinic of Sacramento, California, is now using
   ultrasound treatment to stimulate the kidney cells to reproduce faster and restore deteriorating kidney function.
   It is possible that this therapeutic capability is available
   where you live.)

3. Gout may develop from the abundance of uric acid in the system. So may recurrent and painful arthritis attacks that often last for hours.
4. Depression and other emotional conditions are not uncommon to fasters along with development of anemia and low thyroid function.
5. Hair loss is temporary in most cases but permanent in others.
6. Muscle cramping and spasms are common in fasting, making the experience unpleasant to painful.
7. Generalized malnutrition is common, but can usually be corrected later with proper supplementation. (Patients are often not conscientious in following through on such a rebuilding program and can then be subject to a host of illnesses.)
8. Lean tissue is lost along with fat, and the rebuilding program takes time in order for the person involved to feel restored to full good health.
9. Mild exercise such as slow walking supervised by hospital personnel can be performed, but exertion beyond that level often produces dizziness and possible collapse and injury, as well as heart arrhythmias, which could contribute to heart attack and even death.

There is the case for and against total fasting. Some experts in the field think fasting is almost as dangerous as major surgery and taking powerful drugs. This is why so many of them prefer to administer a low-calorie diet to patients, along with heavy vitamin, mineral, and amino acid supplements as a measure to prevent serious complications.

To fast or not to fast? That is the question—a question that can be answered only by the obese or otherwise seriously overweight individual.

Many authorities feel that a more moderate approach can accomplish most things that a total fast can, particularly if the patient can manage to defeat the body's stubbornly resisting setpoint.

This can be done!

HOW TO BEAT THE STUBBORN SETPOINT

Every man that striveth for the mastery is temperate in all things . . . I Corinthians 9:25 (KJV)

A WISE guy once said, "I believe in moderation even in moderation."

This extremist philosophy undoubtedly led him to overeat and underexercise, and consequently he was overweight and probably obese, following one crash diet after another.

At first crash diets seem to work. Then they begin to work you over. Intemperately low-calorie food intake triggers the setpoint—your obstinate archenemy against losing weight, a built-in biochemical mechanism that protects the body against starvation and a survival system that automatically lowers the metabolic rate, the rate at which food is burned in the cells.

So, how can you outwit this compensatory mechanism that cannot distinguish between a self-imposed diet and the threat of starvation?

First, don't decrease your caloric intake radically. A 600- to 800-calorie diet will only serve to jangle all the alarm bells, whereas a gradual decrease in food intake will not as readily let the setpoint know what's going on.

Some authorities state that fat foods alert the setpoint even when total calories are not sharply decreased. Other authorities don't even believe there is a setpoint. Whatever they choose to call it, a biochemical regulator does exist to make us burn our food fuel more economically when it senses a decline in dietary intake. A setpoint is a setpoint is a setpoint, Gertrude.

A certain perverseness exists in the setpoint. One of my amply proportioned biochemist friends comments sadly: "The best way to gain weight is to cut calories."

Exaggeration? Not really. Like a marked decrease in caloric intake, a skipped meal serves as a trigger to the setpoint that starvation is about to set in. Then just try to lose weight! Furthermore, when you skip meals or sharply reduce your intake of calories, you are more likely to binge.

Weight loss expert Wayne Callaway, director for the Center for Clinical Nutrition at George Washington University in Washington, D.C., claims to have a formula for losing weight without opposition from the setpoint. Follow a daily diet of 10 calories for each pound you carry around—for example: 10 calories times 130 pounds or 1300 calories—combined with 20 minutes of vigorous, sustained aerobic exercise.

The setpoint does not appear to battle against calories lost through exercise, so various authorities agree with Dr. Callaway that a moderate reduction in daily calories plus brisk exercising constitutes an effective weight reduction program. Certain experts, such as Dr. Grant Gwinup have conducted experiments showing that exercise alone, that is, spirited exercise for sixty minutes a day, will bring about slow, steady, and enduring weight loss.

Studies and experiments have been carried out all over the world to penetrate the mysteries of why some of us have so much difficulty staying or becoming slender. Out of the fog some fragments of answers are beginning to emerge.

Not long ago, Dr. Albert J. Stunkard, psychiatrist at the University of Pennsylvania School of Medicine and world-renowned authority on weight loss, published an article in the *Journal of The American Medical Association* (JAMA) to the effect that overweight in most instances is caused by a flaw in the genes. He states that our genes exert their influence "across the whole range of body fatness from very thin to very fat."

There you have it. If the genes fit, put them on.

Despite the Stunkard pronouncement, which offers a cop-out for individuals who refuse to do anything about their overweight except read books about overweight, the fact remains that many people succeed with weight loss regimens.

Besides, nobody—including Dr. Stunkard—knows exactly what kind of a mixture genes, diet, and exercise will make. Apparently some latitude exists within our genetic programming so that most of us women won't end up looking like artist Peter Paul Rubens' well-upholstered ladies. The Stunkard discovery makes me feel thankful that I selected my parents and grandparents well.

Another key bit of information coming out of the fog explains how heavyweights and the obese are triggered to overeat. The conventional ways are by an empty stomach, a low blood sugar level, a biochemical nudge by the brain's hypothalamus, and powerfully motivating external cues. Now Jules Hirsch, Irving Faust, and Rudolph Leibel, three brilliant obesity researchers at Rockefeller University, have uncovered the fact that in heavy persons fat cells actually transmit the signal to overeat through the central nervous system.

You are wonderfully made—all of the 60 to 70 trillion cells that are you. And these cells raise a subliminal fuss when they sense that you're not feeding them enough, particularly when you're on a crash diet! However, with God's adaptability created in you, you have metabolic machinery that slows down when you're on any diet, but especially when it's a drastic one.

Under such circumstances you might manifest fatigue or feel cold in temperatures in which you were formerly comfortable; your thinking and remembering could lose some of their sharpness; and you could be anxious or depressed.

Crash diets are self-defeating, as the following illustration shows. Once the body is aware of the madness you are attempting, it says to the setpoint, "Hey, cut the rate of metabolism." So the metabolism slows up to make certain that, by conservation, your body can survive such a siege of deprivation.

Inasmuch as few of us can survive such Spartan torture permanently, you eventually go back to your normal caloric intake— say, 2200 calories. Now your body's thermostat has been set to burn up 900 calories. So you have a surplus of 1300 calories over what your metabolism is geared to handle. Where do these calories go? You guessed it. To all the old familiar places as fat. Sure, the metabolism eventually comes into balance and burns faster and hotter, but first you gain back all the fat you lost in your martyrdom. So does martyrdom pay off? Not in the weight loss league.

But the damage can't be measured solely in terms of calories. If you pursued a regular exercise program along with the low-cal diet, you undoubtedly lost more than just fat: you lost some muscle and other protein tissue. You came out of this with a poor exchange. You lost fat, muscle, and other protein, and you gained back fat only—that is, unless you continued your exercise.

James Braly, M.D., introduced earlier, tells of the meager returns from titanic dieting in two studies. Of 200 individuals in a hospital-controlled setting, 50 percent lost an average of sixty-two pounds, 25 percent averaged a ninety-pound loss, and 38 percent ended up within 30 percent of their ideal weight. However, within several years, more than 95 percent of them had settled back to their uncomfortable, fat-enclosed weight.

Another group of volunteers subjected themselves for three months to a grueling diet of half their usual calories. What did they get for their agony? An average loss of 10 to 20 percent before any more excess poundage refused to budge. Then with the diet's end, they gorged on 5000 calories daily. Soon their weight settled down to the former figure, and they stopped eating voraciously. They, too, had lost fat and protein and gained back fat.

All sorts of fascinating facts about fat have been revealed by the Rockefeller University trio of Hirsch, Faust, and Leibel. One is that obese individuals are not necessarily limited to the inventory of fat cells with which they were born. They can even add fat cells.

So that you can visualize exactly what this means, just imagine that fat cells are like microscopic rubber balloons. As more fat is tucked into them, they inflate. So do you along with them. Obese test subjects have as many as 75 billion fat cells, compared with a normal weight's 27 billion.

Once you have fat cells, you can never lose them; you can only reduce them in size. The Rockefeller University researchers have found the reason people are unable to lose weight in specific parts of the body, such as the hips and thighs in women. Leibel states that fat cells have two kinds of receptors on their surface: alpha and beta. Alpha receptors accumulate fat and beta receptors break it down. Alpha receptors are far more numerous than the beta type on women's hips and thighs, so fat storage occurs much faster than the fat can be broken down.

On the basis of this information, can anything be done to help women who have too much of a good thing on their hips and thighs? Not yet, responds Leibel. There's no quick fix. The Rockefeller team still needs to learn hundreds of answers regarding the conduct of receptors and fat cells.

Speaking of fat cells and outwitting the setpoint, Hirsch offers three secrets to losing weight, secrets so simple they are foolproof: "Eat less, exercise more, and stay with this program for the rest of your life." Yet most individuals will continue seeking an easy fix instead of following a program like this that really works.

New experiments from the Rockefeller University research team indicate that, as demonstrated by the setpoint, the body not only protects us from starvation, but works to stabilize us at a certain weight. In other words, as the following example will illustrate, the body also does its best to keep us from gaining too much, but it appears to be more effective in preventing weight loss.

A young student volunteer agreed to live for a year in a ward room at Rockefeller University to take part in a Hirsch–Leibel experiment.

At the experiment's beginning, he weighed 190 pounds, a normal weight for his height, and required 2850 calories daily to maintain his weight. Of this amount, 183 calories were found to be needed in burning up the food he consumed.

Early in the experiment, he gained twenty pounds, all encircling his waist. It was difficult for him to gain and keep on the excess weight, which made him feel uncomfortable. Then Hirsch and Leibel determined his caloric needs and discovered that he now needed 4620 calories daily just to maintain his weight, and 569 of these calories were necessary to burn up his food. He was like a furnace in need of stoking. Calories were burning up furiously, especially right after meals.

Next the researchers asked him to diet until he could move his weight down to 20 percent under normal. Now his racing metabolism slowed down to a walk. He required only 2871 calories to maintain the lower weight, and only 109 of them were utilized for burning his food.

Exactly what did these contrasting figures show? That when a body is gaining weight, it burns up surplus food at an increasing rate; but when it loses weight, it needs very few calories to burn up food. The experiment demonstrated that the setpoint, or the body's metabolism, works in both directions: It adjusts metabolism to correct any deviation from what is its ideal weight. Another student now going through the same experimental exercise is following the identical biochemical pattern as the first student.

In the realm of weight loss there has long been curiosity as to what happens to the setpoint when people continue to gain and lose weight. Kelly Brownell, at the University of Pennsylvania, found this reaction to what is called "the yo-yo syndrome."

Immediately, he found that people who had been on numerous weight loss diets responded poorly to his weight reduction program. In collaboration with M.R.C. Greenwood, of Vassar College, Brownell conducted a rat experiment that revealed that the lab animals on yo-yo diets became food-efficient.

During a second time on the same weight reduction diet, the rats dropped weight at only half the rate as on the first diet. Allowed to regain weight after their second dieting program, they regained weight three times faster than they had after their first weight reduction. Brownell believes they were defending their ideal body weight.

Still another researcher, George Blackburn of the Harvard Medical School, has found that human subjects follow the same pattern as that of rats in yo-yo dietary programs. In his metabolic ward the extremely obese come to live in an insolated environment and shed weight on a carefully controlled, very low calorie diet.

Blackburn has found that people who return to his ward three or four times find it ever more difficult to lose weight. So yo-yo dieting makes a person use food more efficiently and increases the difficulty in subsequent dieting efforts.

However, there's more to the weight reduction story than just the setpoint. You can put out energy in three distinct ways: 1) basal metabolism (the speed and efficiency at which you burn up food in your cells when you are at the resting level); 2) thermogenesis (energy expressed as heat given off at a metabolic rate above the resting level); 3) physical activity.

Expressed in bald terms, basal metabolism describes the efficiency of the thyroid gland. Food-induced thermogenesis (another form of thermogenesis is being exposed to environmental temperatures below body temperature) comes in two packages: obligatory and regulatory. Obligatory thermogenesis is the energy cost of digesting, absorbing, and converting nutrients for immediate use or for storage; regulatory thermogenesis is energy expenditure for physical and mental activity.

A central part of the thermogenesis process is brown fat, a very unusual kind of adipose tissue that collects below the neck and goes down the back like a small mat. No two persons are endowed with the same amount of brown fat or with brown fat of equal capability. Individuals who have a small amount have far more difficulty staying slender than those who have inherited a large amount. However, people whose brown fat functions inefficiently come out on the short end, too.

Let's check into what brown fat is and does. First, it's different from white fat that accumulates under the skin, acting as insulation that has a way of gathering into unsightly bulges and staying there.

The mat of brown fat is located deeper in the body and is bound to the skeleton. Its brown coloring comes from a multitude of infinitesimal biochemical powerhouses known as mitochondria and cytochromes. These energy-producing cell parts are mini-furnaces that generate body heat and burn up superfluous calories. Only about 10 to 20 percent of total body fat is brown fat. The remaining 80 to 90 percent is the white stuff that does us little good and could do us much harm.

Brown fat is heat-generating, and when you pig out at a party or on Thanksgiving, Christmas, or New Year's, it does you the favor of burning off as many excess calories as possible. After an overindulgence at times like these, you probably experienced such an abundance of body heat that you couldn't sleep. So you tossed and turned and wrestled with the bedding all night, not realizing that your brown fat was doing you a favor by trying to compensate for your overindulgence. Your brown fat wasn't deliberately ruining your sleep, it was just trying to normalize your weight.

How bears are able to hibernate and maintain steady high temperatures despite winter's cold offers a clue as to why fat is burned off so readily when human beings perform exercises in a cold environment. Bears are endowed with a large supply of brown fat. Cold temperatures act as a signal for their thermostat to keep heat production high.

An article in *The Physician And Sports Medicine* describes a rather unique experiment. Seven lightly clad men (shorts, T-shirts, socks, gym shoes, and light cotton gloves) exercised for an hour each on a cycle ergometer at two different temperatures: 10°C and 22°C. The researchers discovered that total energy use increased by 13 percent and—get this!—fat utilization was 35 percent higher when test subjects exercised in the cold for 60 minutes. The conclusion? Cold and exercise have an additive effect on fat utilization.

Biochemist Jeffrey Bland, Ph.D., asserts that to get the setpoint working for you, you have to activate the brown fat, which has a tendency to become less responsive to extra calories as we grow older. We can't sit around watching ourselves adding fat as the brown fat mechanism grows less effective. Let's find ways to stimulate the brown fat. This can be done, and we can do it with certain nutrient supplements. (Restricting calories is just one way of attacking the weight loss problem.)

Accenting certain positive measures and eliminating certain negatives can encourage the brown fat to start burning hot again. A supplement of linoleic-acid-rich essential fatty acids (EFAs) has been found to rev up the metabolism of fat. Evening primrose oil and black currant oil, available at nutrition centers, can also stimulate the brown fat.

Can't we get enough EFAs from the conventional polyunsaturated oils—corn, peanut, safflower, sunflower seed, and wheat germ? Not necessarily. Some oils are not biologically active. Others are processed for cooking fat and margarine, losing their EFA activity and even possibly becoming anti-EFA factors.

EFAs are precursors to prostaglandins, key short-term regulators that help control all body organs. Without enough EFAs, numerous physical abnormalities occur: serious malfunction of the heart and circulatory defects; acne and eczema; subnormal immune function; wounds that fail to heal; shortcomings or failure of reproduction (mainly in men); inflammatory ailments and arthritis; fat liver and fibrosis; failure of the brain to develop properly; imbalance of body water; and atrophy of the ducted glands.

Western lifestyle practices and products block a person from translating linoleic acid to gamma-linoleic acid (GLA) and dihomo-gamma-linoleic acid (DGLA). Among these practices and products are: a heavy intake of saturated fats and cholesterol; processed vegetable oil; refined sugar; steroids and birth control pills; alcohol; virus infections; degenerative diseases; radiation, and zinc deficiency.

Until recent years, it was thought that mother's milk was the only source of GLA and DGLA. Then the exciting properties of evening primrose oil (Efamol) were discovered. This oil is pressed from the seeds of the evening primrose, a beautiful, yellow wildflower of the eastern seaboard that blossoms and dies in one evening. Evening primrose oil contains 8 to 9 percent GLA and 70-plus percent cis-linoleic acid, the EFA-active form.

One thing leads to another with evening primrose oil. Its experimental use for psychiatric purposes by Dr. K.S. Vaddadi in England led to the discovery that some patients gained an unexpected bonus—they lost appreciable weight. Noting this, heavyset nurses took evening primrose capsules and lost weight, too.

This serendipitous occurrence brought about a study of evening primrose oil for weight reduction. Obese and less heavy test subjects seemed to get the best results. Among patients more than 10 percent overweight who took the evening primrose oil supplement, 50 percent lost significant poundage without even changing their diet, and they reported a reduced appetite.

Evening primrose oil and black currant oil—a more recent product also high in linoleic acid—are thought to stimulate the brown fat back into full service. Deficiencies of vitamins A, C, and E, Beta carotene (a vitamin A precursor), vitamins B-3 and B-6, and biotin, as well as zinc and magnesium, essential amino acids, and, most important, EFAs, reduce efficiency of brown fat function.

A study of women 26 to 67 years old who failed to lose weight on various diets, or who could not keep it off if they did, concluded that the women had thermogenically unresponsive brown fat, mainly due to insufficiency of their thyroid function. The thyroid, shaped like a butterfly or small bow tie, sits inside the base of the neck. When the patients' hypothyroidism (low thyroid function) was treated with thyroid hormones, brown fat became activated and generated heat.

This isn't always the solution, however. Recently it was discovered that when the thyroid gland is functioning well, another problem is often present. The liver and muscle tissues sometimes cannot convert the thyroid-secreted hormones into active hormones that affect the basal metabolic rate.

Preventive medicine specialists sometimes correct this condition with daily supplements of 15 to 30 milligrams of zinc and 3 to 10 milligrams of copper.

Still another way to stimulate the heat-producing factory of brown fat is through meals made up of complex carbohydrates, moderate protein, and low fat.

Of course, exercise is the most effective way of getting the kind of action you want out of your distribution of brown fat. More about exercise is coming up.

NONEXERCISING: THE SIN OF OMISSION

. . . And be sure your sin will find you out.   Numbers
32:23 (KJV)

*T*HE only physical activity performed by some heavyweights
is exercising their imagination, picking up options, and running through the mail.

That's not going to lose unwanted pounds!

The missing dimension in most weight control regimens is
EXERCISE! This word deserves tall capital letters. It is that important.

True, the Bible gives little attention to exercise, undoubtedly
because when men from Abraham to Jesus needed to get from
here to there, they walked fifteen to twenty miles a day and
thought nothing of it. They performed every sort of manual labor.
Ninety-five percent of the work in those days was physical. Now
only about 5 percent of the work is physical.

Underexercising contributes more to excessive weight than
overeating. So indicates a joint report by two federal government
departments: Health and Human Services and Agriculture.

Some 32 million 25- to 74-year-old Americans are overweight
and 11.7 million are obese. Related findings disclose that obesity
is more common among the poor—those below the poverty
level—and among black women than among other socioeconomic
groups.

The report does some finger pointing at the unusually heavy

consumption of fat by Americans—approximately 41 percent of the diet—as a second major cause of overweight and obesity and its accompanying physical disorders.

Another federal government report shatters a common misconception about weight gain: that middle-age spread is caused by getting older. Metabolism keeps slowing down and weight keeps picking up.

Physiologist Carol N. Meredith, of the U.S. Department of Agriculture's Human Nutrition Research Center on Aging at Tufts University in Boston, says it's not middle age that determines body fat levels. It is the decreasing number of hours that individuals devote to aerobic exercise. The amount of spirited physical activity also determines the caloric needs and aerobic capacity, a measure of fitness determined by the amount of oxygen used per minute.

"It's generally assumed that as people get older, something changes biologically to cause them to add fat and lose physical fitness and that exercise can't alter this trend," Meredith says, "However, a few studies indicate otherwise."

To differentiate between the effects of aging and decreased physical activity, she and associates compared the fitness level and exercise habits of twelve extremely active men—half of them in their twenties and half in their fifties. All of them had been cycling, rowing, and running regularly for a minimum of two years.

According to Meredith, "Their fat level had nothing to do with their age—only with the amount of time they spent exercising."

Meredith admits that the study had too few subjects to warrant making sweeping claims. However, the findings were definite and clear-cut. As an example, one 54-year-old man who ran fourteen hours a week had the same percent of body fat as a 19-year old who also trained fourteen hours a week.

Yet the middle-aged men, as a group, had 77 percent more body fat than the young men, "because they exercised fewer hours—seven and a half per week compared with twelve and a half for the young men. Meredith states, "Time is the important factor."

After twelve hours per week of exercise, fat reduction becomes less marked, Meredith observes. Also, the middle-aged men had 15 percent less aerobic capacity and needed 17 percent fewer calories to maintain their weight despite their higher fat level.

Both groups had the same metabolic rate and nearly the same lean muscle mass. In order to be aerobic, exercise has to be sustained for more than twenty minutes and involve large groups of muscles—for instance, brisk walking, cycling, rowing, and running. Weight lifting, which targets specific muscle groups, is not aerobic.

Aging itself seems to reduce voluntary movement, Meredith admits. Scientists have observed this occurrence in animals and in primitive societies where sedentary jobs and "too little time" are not factors. The reason for age-related inertia is not known.

Every person in the study but one started exercising regularly during adolescence, leading Meredith to conclude, "It's possible that a habit of vigorous exercise is easier to maintain if it is initiated in early age."

This is a problem. Despite the present physical fitness craze, the vast majority of young people are still on the sidelines—worse, in the TV easy chair. That's the reason that the middle-age spread is no longer a monopoly of the middle-aged.

Regular, spirited exercise may burn off surplus fat better than dieting. At least one important authority thinks so. Grant Gwinup, M.D., professor of metabolism and endocrinology at the University of California at Irvine, maintains that his program of vigorous bicycle riding helps even heavy individuals lose weight regularly without dieting. He explains:

"For getting rid of excess weight, exercising is far more effective than dieting. If you exercise just 30 minutes or more daily without dieting, you lose fat and keep muscle, which is the name of the game."

New studies reveal that dynamic, big-muscle exercises such as running and bicycling generate metabolic rates that are eight to ten times resting values. Vigorous physical activity often raises the resting metabolic rate for up to fifteen hours after exercise—an important argument for exercise as a giant key to efficient weight loss.

In recent years exercise has been recognized as an effective means of losing or stabilizing weight. Previously it was thought that exercise would increase appetite to the point where the caloric input would nullify or exceed caloric output. And it was believed that calorie burning by moderate exercise was negligible in comparison with what could be done by fasting or semistarvation.

The encouraging truth is that regular exercise can indeed make a significant inroad to getting rid of stored fat. A recently discovered fact is that daily physical activity is necessary for good functioning of the feeding control biomechanism. Individuals who sit in chairs all day at work or at leisure do not receive the benefit of a finely-tuned balance between energy output and food intake.

Inability to regulate food intake, paired with minimal physical activity, seems to account for "creeping obesity" in industrialized societies. For individuals who are physically active, appetite is in a reactive zone where it is easier to match calories of food intake with the daily expenditure of energy.

Certainly physical exercise exerts a powerful influence on fat melting. Let's look at the above sentence in reverse. Inactivity contributes to weight gain. If this were not so, why are geese and pigs penned in and permitted to gorge themselves before being sent to market? Why are cattle transported from the open range to feedlots and overfed before being marketed?

If physical activity weren't so important in regulating weight, why did the National Research Council formulate its Recommended Daily Allowances (RDAs) on that basis?

A 2400-calorie intake was planned for physically inactive men, 4500 calories for very active men, and up to 6000 calories for heavy laborers: farmers, field soldiers, lumberjacks, miners, and athletes. Lumberjacks and endurance athletes (marathon runners and cross-country skiers) are usually greyhound lean despite their rich caloric intake. Obviously, their extreme food intake is needed just to meet requirements of training and has no relation to accumulation of body fat.

Consider a fascinating study of 200 patients by James H. Greene, M.D., of Iowa City, Iowa, regarding physical activity as a stabilizer of weight.

All the patients became obese when the following drastic life changes stopped their physical activities short: the shift to a sedentary occupation, going blind, or being disabled in a serious car accident.

Even partial inactivity appears to contribute more to obesity than overeating. Dr. Jean Mayer and Dr. Mary Louise Johnson studied the food intake and physical activity of two distinct categories of obese high school girls: those who ate slightly fewer calories and exercised far less than normal-weights, and a small segment of outgoing, happy obese girls who ate more than the normal-weights and exercised just as much. Exercise made the latter group more muscular and less plump in appearance.

In another Mayer study obese and normal-weight children, matched for age and social status, were filmed during such sports activities as swimming, tennis, and volleyball. The obese moved only a fraction as much as those of normal weight and expended much less energy.

Still another Mayer experiment again showed the strong influence of exercise on weight loss. Obese and normal-weight boys were observed in mandatory physical activity and in eating. Normal-weight boys ate more and gained some poundage. However, obese boys ate only a little more and lost weight.

A rarely realized fact about weight loss is that the obese and even the moderately overweight can melt off unwanted poundage more efficiently than normal-weights. In the process of exercising, the obese burn up more fat than normal-weights because their movements are impaired and often cumbersome, and so require more energy.

Likewise, a person 20 percent overweight can burn away more pounds than a normal-weight performing the identical exercise, inasmuch as accumulated fat makes the activity more clumsy and inefficient.

Are you 20 percent overweight? Do you exercise regularly and with vigor? If so, you're going to win at weight loss and gain some rewards: a sense of accomplishment, additional self-esteem, and optimism for even greater weight loss.

All right, enough generalizations. How about some specifics such as, "What are the best fat-melting exercises?"

Nothing fancy. "Stationary bike riding is the best calorie burner, with moving bicycle riding, running, jogging, and brisk walking following in that order," says Dr. Grant Gwinup, on the basis of many of his own research projects.

Now, stationary bike riding doesn't mean using one of those electrically powered bikes that does all the work while you go along for the ride. The bike has no weight to lose.

Where does swimming come in relative to weight loss? It doesn't. Gwinup conducted an experiment to compare weight loss among moderately obese, healthy, young women eager to burn off fat by means of daily exercise instead of dieting. They were randomly assigned to brisk walking, stationary bike riding, or swimming. During a twenty-eight-week period, the women became better conditioned and upped their exercise time from five to sixty minutes daily. The walkers dropped 11 percent of their original weight; the cyclists lost 13 percent; and the swimmers lost nothing. Actually, the swimmers gained 3 percent.

So far as the swimmers were concerned, Gwinup attempts to explain the mystery:

"The body's natural defense mechanism against cold is hoarding fat. I suspect that's the reason. Some of the world's fattest people are eskimos. Then, too, Polynesians, who spend a great deal of time in the water, are also fat. Japanese women pearl divers swim for hours each day and they are fat but fit."

Another part of the answer could come from an experiment I read about not long ago. It could be that swimming creates a greater need for food than other sports activities. Women in swim training took in about 15 percent more calories in training and competition than did collegiate tennis players.

Your effectiveness in burning fat depends on three factors: 1) how strenuously you exercise; 2) how long you exercise; and 3) your weight.

Exercises that melt off fat best involve using large muscle mass, muscle contraction, and gross movement of the body to another place. If you pursue such exercises and still aren't losing much, or any, weight, it may be that your sessions haven't been long enough. Don't become discouraged and quit. Increase your time at the activity.

Another experiment by Dr. Gwinup illustrates this need. While remaining on their usual diet, eleven obese women increased their time at daily walking for more than a year. Not a single one of them could lose until she began walking more than thirty minutes at a time. These women dropped an average of twenty-two pounds each in a year of fast walking and maintained their loss for another year.

Still another experiment reveals that amount of time spent performing the exercise is of great importance. Three groups of men exercised for twenty weeks, each group walking and running for a set time: fifteen, thirty, or forty-five minutes daily. The results were compared with those of a nonactive control group.

All three groups lost body fat, skinfolds, and waist girth in comparison with the controls. However, the 45-minute group lost the most, particularly body fat.

Sometimes individuals become discouraged when each ounce of fat leaves reluctantly. Gwinup states that that is exactly how weight should go off—slowly. "A pound a week is just about right," he says. "If it goes much faster, you'll be losing only water and muscle and important minerals and other nutrients important to your health."

Rather than be satisfied with slow and solid progress, many people who are physically unable to exercise as long at a stretch as they would like tend to quit with a remark such as, "I guess I'm getting too old for this."

A doctor's checkup could readily determine if that remark is valid. However, in most instances the individuals involved just haven't given themselves time to build up. As yet, nobody is selling a product they sorely need: instant patience.

Really, it's never too late to start unless you think it is. Let me cite an example that's dear to my heart.

Dr. Herbert DeVries, of the University of Southern California School of Medicine, accepted the challenge of supervising a moderate, fifteen-minute daily exercise session for men from a retirement colony—52- to 88-year-olds.

Of course, he started them slowly, but within several months they all showed remarkable transformations. They lost flab and weight and developed 35 percent more breathing capacity, a 30 percent increase in ability to deliver oxygen to the cells, improved ability to sleep soundly, and release from nervous tension, aggression, anger, frustration, and hostility. They also experienced well-being and showed a far more youthful appearance.

It was tough getting started, however, because so many of the men had become sedentary, with bodies accustomed to staying that way. Nobody said it would be easy. And it may not be so for you for reasons beyond plain inertia. Conditions and events are not arranged in your favor. You have to rearrange them. Society lets you know by sight and sound how it worships the slender body. Yet it tempts and tortures you with seductive ads for gooey desserts swimming in chocolate syrup and topped with whipping cream, and then it keeps you from burning off unwanted fat with at-home and at-work laborsaving devices.

So-called civilization is separating us even farther from nature—from our connectedness with God. One of my friends with quite a few miles on his odometer wraps this idea up nicely in the following words:

"A few generations ago, almost everybody worked outside. I mean, they worked physically. Now we are in the Exerciseless Age and indoors, working mostly with our minds instead of our muscles. We have desk jobs, to which we drive in cars. Power steering, power brakes and automatic transmission take away the need for physical effort.

"Our workplaces have elevators or escalators, telephones and intercoms. In sports, we are mainly spectators—in the stands or in front of the TV. Everything is so easy for us that we work hard creating physical activities to replace those which have been eliminated."

As in the workplace, we have laborsaving and step-saving devices at home: telephone extension cords, multiple phones, portable units, and car phones. Paradoxically, the golfer who plays for fun and exercise drives around the eighteen holes in a battery-powered cart.

Everywhere you look around the house is a mechanical or electrical slave: electric hedge clipper, power lawn mower, power edge trimmer, tractor lawn mower, snow blower, electric carving knives, cream whipper, blender, juicer, food processor, toaster, waffle maker, percolator, electric refrigerator, electric toothbrush, shoe polisher, automatic garage door opener.

Some of these mechanical and electrical slaves will have to be freed if you seriously want to lose weight. You may have to shift from labor saving to labor spending. Everything you do yourself burns some calories. Don't save steps. Take them. Walk fast. (Beware of lonely, dark places for your evening exercise. One of my acquaintances really got "exercised" by some toughs.)

Stand rather than sit while dressing if your equilibrium is okay. (If it isn't, don't try it, please.) Wash and wax your own car if your pride and status permit. Charge into your housework and yard work with enthusiasm and energy. The more active you are, the more calories you will burn. Forget about the remote-control TV channel selector. Move to your TV to change channels, instead of into High Calorie Country: your kitchen.

Because I enjoy doing the things I'm recommending, I can lose at least half a pound weekly in these ways. You can, too.

Choreographer Jean Martin, of Atherton, California, who has danced in films including Fred Astaire's "Blue Skies," performs simple, calorie-burning exercises while watching TV. (The frequency of each exercise is just the suggested amount. Well-conditioned individuals may wish to continue as long as they like.)

Her "TVehicle" exercise involves becoming a bicycle while watching television programs that require no concentration. (Do any of them?) Lie on your back, pull in your abdomen, and draw your knees toward you as in bicycling. Do this ten times with each leg.

"Doggone" is another of Jean's pets. Just get your hands on the floor like feet, as a dog stands. Pull in your right knee toward your chest, then stretch your right leg back far behind you. Do the same with your left leg. Repeat ten times with each leg. Jean sometimes does this fifty times with each leg, but by then she's dog tired.

Her last TV exercise is the "Sweet Roll." Stand with your feet slightly apart and bend, keeping your back parallel with floor. Keep your chin up to watch the program even if you are the best entertainment in the room. Bend your right knee and roll in that direction. Then do the same thing to the left side. Do ten from each side.

Jean has a few telephone exercises to accompany long talkers.

Sit in a backed chair, tighten up your tummy, and then do leg lifts, right then left and then together, ten each. Another phone exercise is gently raising your knees, one at a time, toward your chest. (Jean didn't warn about this, but it's my advice not to exercise too vigorously. This could cause heavy breathing. Remember, you're on the phone!)

Another friend, Gene Arceri, writes celebrity books, the best known of which is *Red*, the biography of Susan Hayward. He doesn't like formal exercise, so he walks the most challenging hills of San Francisco daily, refusing to drive a car, take a bus, or ride the little cable cars (". . . halfway to the stars").

If you don't have hills like San Francisco's in your home city, make do with what you have and no grumbling, please. Or move to the "City by the Bay." Those who don't have hills walk barefooted and briskly along the wet sands of the beach or on the dry sands of the desert. It is best to do the desert bit early in the morning, not by the heat of the day. Remember, "Mad dogs and Englishmen go out in the noonday sun." Wear shoes if you do walk in the heat of the day.

If you don't have a beach or a desert handy, please don't tug at my sleeve for another option. Just walk fast and long on your flat, unsandy cement sidewalks and be wary of any raised slabs! (Or sue the city for whiplash!)

It isn't always necessary to perform strenuous or grueling exercises to see yourself diminish to the point where you're satisfied with yourself. Increased physical activity in the light to moderate range—just above the sedentary—often depresses appetite and consequently lowers food intake, as studies show.

Experiments with animals also demonstrate that this principle works—works wonders. Sedentary animals motivated to exercise for an hour a day begin eating appreciably less.

In a study done in the industrial area of West Bengal, India, individuals asked to perform moderate to heavy labor increased their caloric intake in proportion to the difficulty of their work. Even at that, their body weight remained well below that of the sedentary laborer. Persons assigned light physical activity showed a lower intake of food than the sedentary workers, and lower weight, as well.

Of importance to all of us who want to keep our weight

under control, or who want to have less poundage to keep under control, are several studies that show that when young men and women start only a moderate exercise program, they decrease the amount of food eaten daily. As a result, they also begin losing weight.

A bonus value from regular, brisk aerobic exercise is relief from nervous tension and stress, which sometimes underlie over-eating.

DON'T LET STRESS SABOTAGE YOUR DIET

A merry heart doeth good like a medicine, but a broken spirit drieth the bones. Proverbs 17–22 (KJV)

*O*NCE upon a time not too many decades ago, a popular song, "Put On A Happy Face," cheered the nation. Now psychologists tell us that smiling even when you don't feel like it can change things inside you and bring on a positive mood.

Actually, nineteen centuries before there were psychologists, the Bible stated something similar: "A merry heart doeth good like a medicine . . ."

A fascinating study by psychologist Suzanne Kobasa, formerly of the University of Chicago, gives momentum to this Scripture. She found that business executives with a positive, optimistic outlook and a feeling of some control over events adjusted to and withstood stress far better than downbeat, pessimistic, "controlled-by-events" executives, and thus they were better able to avoid illness.

Being pushed around by stressors and the negative emotional responses to them is a major cause of overeating. Therefore, it is important for would-be weight losers to learn how to handle stress before it manhandles them.

Extreme stressors such as a death in the family or being fired from a job usually make individuals stop eating entirely. But milder stress—the little emotional foxes that nibble at us—makes us eat, often unconsciously, when not hungry and scuttles our best intentions and resolutions and the diet based on them.

The worst part of it is, sometimes stressful emotions are so subtle that we are not fully aware of them and the dietary damage they trigger. Then, too, we may be aware of the emotion but not of the fact that it is the cause of our overeating.

A physician friend told me about the case of a woman who, motivated by loneliness, married a domineering man shortly after her first husband died. It turned out to be one of those "repent at leisure" marriages. Within a little more than a year, she had lost her sylph-like figure, rounding out with thirty-four additional pounds.

In tears, she related to the doctor how she had outgained most of her wardrobe and that her husband, a prosperous hardware store owner whose checkbook always seemed hard to open, now refused to buy her anything. "You ate yourself out of your clothes. Now diet yourself back into them," he told her.

The doctor asked her to fill out a questionnaire on a week's typical meals and snacks. It turned out her snacks were the meals and her meals the snacks. And what snacks! Ding-Dongs™, Twinkies™, brownies, donuts, cookies, potato chips, and cokes, among other bad goodies.

Asked why she snacked so heavily, the woman said, "I don't really know. I never had a weight problem before. I even modeled at one time. All I can tell you for sure is that my husband is getting me down. I'm frustrated. He's so domineering, tight with money, and always ridiculing me in front of relatives and friends with remarks such as, 'You have a great figure. There's just too much of it.' "

If she became angry and responded, her husband would explode in a temper tantrum. She never knew if he would hit her, but was always anxious about it. She requested a special diet, but my friend said she wouldn't need one if she followed an appropriate course of action.

"Your overeating is not uncommon under such trying circumstances," he told her. "The fact that your husband ridicules you just compounds the problem."

Then he told her about research done by Dr. Walter Hamburger, professor of psychiatry at the University of Rochester, which had uncovered four categories of life conditions or situations that prompt overeating:

1. Nonspecific emotional tensions.
2. Intolerable life situations.
3. Hidden emotional illness, particularly as an expression of hysteria.
4. A food addiction.

Certainly "intolerable life situations" was the stress category that made her a junk food junkie. The doctor suggested that she get away from it all by visiting her out-of-town parents or other relatives in order to regain emotional stability. Then she would be able to cut calories and begin to lose weight. Upon returning home she could demonstrate to her husband that domestic tranquility and considerate treatment was all she needed for weight control.

She followed the doctor's recommendation, enjoying peace, normal eating, and losing weight so much that she stayed away a week longer than expected. This turned out to be a blessing. Three weeks later when she returned, she found a lonely husband who was delighted to see her and overjoyed about the nine pounds she had lost. In his soft mood, they were able to discuss her problem rationally. Once he understood that he was contributing to her problem, he began cooperating instead of criticizing. You guessed it: a happy ending. She melted her weight down to normal.

Without a doubt, food helps relieve us of pain, whether psychological or physical. Since we were kids, sweets particularly have been associated with a reward for being hurt. A skinned knee was worth a sugar cookie from Mom. The pattern is set early, so that when in adulthood we feel ill-used, blue, or anxious, we tend to reward ourselves with sweets.

A growing body of literature reveals that our emotional state, our certainty or uncertainty in coping with problems, influences the kind of food we seek. Anxious, depressed, unhappy people crave and eat sweets and other junk food. Individuals who feel they have more control over events tend toward more substantial foods.

High-carbohydrate snacks—candy, pastries, chips, french fries—increase the amount of serotonin, a key neurotransmitter in the brain, and bring us a short-term calming effect. Individuals who feel down most of the time habitually eat carbohydrate snacks—do they ever pack the calories!—and give themselves a lift with higher brain levels of serotonin.

In the same manner that snack foods elevate serotonin, so does binge eating or consuming excessive sweets release endorphins, pain-relieving natural opiates.

A study of bulimics by researchers at the University of Wisconsin in Madison verifies that observation. Bulimics' uncontrollable eating binges favor carbohydrates, especially sweets. The Wisconsin scientists discovered higher blood levels of endorphins in bulimics who induce vomiting than in those who do not and in normal individuals.

Psychologist-biochemist Adam Drenowski at the University of Michigan says that stress helps raise the blood levels of endorphins, which in turn appear to heighten the craving for sweets and other carbohydrates. Drenowski thinks this may be why a stressed person "reaches for a box of chocolates."

And many an anxious, frustrated, or depressed homemaker does just that until she gets to the bottom of things. Then, with a sigh, she throws out the candy box and says to herself, "Now that they're gone, I won't be tempted to eat anymore." Somehow, however, another box of chocolates soon appears—a lifeline for the next bout of emotional stress.

Drenowski doesn't have all the answers to the stress-endorphins–"craving for sweets"-binges connection. But neurobiologist Sarah Leibowitz of Rockefeller University has a few clues. Her specialty is finding the relationship of certain brain chemicals—neurotransmitters—to eating preferences. Neurotransmitters are specialized chemical substances that transmit impulses from one nerve cell to another.

Leibowitz has made the breakthrough discovery that certain neurotransmitters regulate our appetite and dictate preferences at a specific time for carbohydrates, fats, or protein, the three major classifications of food. For instance, norepinephrine excites the hunger for carbohydrates. A chemical called neuropeptide Y can make the appetite run wild. This most powerful appetite stimulant causes rats to multiply their intake of food by twelve times, so that they devour twenty-four hours' worth of food in two hours.

Then, too, the kind of foods we eat can influence the type of neurotransmitters produced by the brain and thus the neurotransmitter balance. When the balance is tilted a vicious cycle starts, causing binge eating, which contributes to further brain chemistry chaos.

The neurotransmitter serotonin suppresses the desire for carbohydrate intake, although eating carbohydrates enriches brain levels of serotonin in a backhanded biochemical manner. Low levels of serotonin seem to contribute to depression. Still another neurotransmitter, dopamine, kills the desire for food, particularly proteins.

Certain kinds of emotional overeating come about because people are not always able to distinguish real hunger from anxiety-motivated eating. Psychologist Stanley Schachter says anxious people may often eat to relieve feelings of anxiety.

Do certain personalities and emotional patterns make individuals prone to become overweight? Yes.

The U.S. Public Health Service sponsored a three-year study of personality and emotions relative to overweight, in which Drs. Benjamin Kotkov, Stanley S. Kanter, and Joseph Rosenthal of the Boston Dispensary of the New England Medical Center, questioned and tested 135 overweight women as well as a control group of 80 normal-weight women. By means of multiple psychological techniques, they unearthed revealing emotional traits.

Overweight women were found to be far more repressed than the normal-weights—more anxious, tense, and tending to hold anger inside. Repressed anger encourages depression. Another of their marked characteristics was that they appeared preoccupied with themselves, not looking for or encouraging new social relationships. They just tolerated social life, were tense, uncomfortable, and often miserable, especially in meeting new people. Certain ones were ill at ease in their clothing. Whether or not the test subjects were moderately or extremely overweight, married or single, educated or uneducated, moderate or high IQ, they all revealed a similar constellation of neurotic traits.

Related studies following this one reveal other emotional

traits that motivate people to overeat: boredom, frustration at a stalled career, and, among many others, working day-in and day-out in a hated job.

In his early days of prominence, when he wrote the book *The Stress of Life*, Dr. Hans Selye observed that people who are bored or even dissatisfied with their employment or their social relations are compelled to find consolation in whatever offers comfort. That "whatever" is often food.

As certain circumstances and situations may induce a person to drink, they may also compel others to overeat. This is what Dr. Selye calls "the principle of deviation." Plainly, some people eat because they have nothing better to do or to substitute for doing something better.

In some instances, obesity may be a badge of stress, particularly in response to continued, relentlessly frustrating experience. Obesity and the deformity it creates compound this frustration, bringing on more excessive eating and with it the distinct possibility of cardiovascular complications and diabetes.

Selye says that overeating does more than just bring gratification in compensation for emotional abuse experienced. It also draws blood away from the brain, giving rise to a soothing effect that makes the situation more tolerable.

Richard B. Stuart and Barbara Davis, weight control authorities, claim that cues to overeat come not only from the outside but also from the inside—from such emotions as depression, an emotional state noted for stimulating overeating.

Don't for a minute think that depression is caused only by external circumstances—delays, financial disasters, career blockage, being unappreciated, disappointment in love, or fifty-seven other varieties of frustration. Biochemical stresses from ill-conceived, nutrient-deficient weight loss diets invite depression, too, and with it more overeating—of the wrong things.

Unfortunately, many individuals who follow weight loss diets are concerned only with shedding excess poundage rather than with losing weight while at the same time nourishing themselves.

Low-calorie diets, notoriously short of the vitamin B complex, are tailor-made to bring on emotional stress. Several studies have shown that subnutritional, imbalanced diets endured by prisoners of war transform normal, even-natured men into morbid, depressed, anxious, irritable, trigger-tempered, and twisted versions of themselves.

Think what vitamin- and mineral-deficient diets can do to those already overweight and depressed! Refined sugars and starches are pseudofoods, which deplete the limited intake of B vitamins in typical American meals.

Vitamin B-1 (thiamin) is often called "the morale vitamin" because it contributes to making your nervous system and thus your emotional life stable. It is essential to food assimilation and digestion—(mainly sugars, starches, and alcohol)—to the secretion of hydrochloric acid in the stomach (an important aid to proper digestion), and to sound muscle tone in the stomach, intestines, and heart.

Most Americans run a vitamin B-1 deficit because they fail to eat the few foods that contain them: wheat germ and bran and rice polish. All of these are milled away, in food processing as shown in chapter 5, "Imitation Foods for Real People."

Unless you get thiamin from whole grain cereals or breads, you will have to derive it from food supplements such as blackstrap molasses, bran, brewer's yeast, rice polishings, or wheat germ, or from the vitamin supplement itself.

Excessive refined sugar, alcohol, and smoking steal the small amount of existing vitamin B-1, leaving you at a deficit for handling its stabilizing functions mentioned above. Then a vitamin B-1-impoverished diet aggravates the emotions, leaving you irritable, blue, or deep in the well of depression.

So what do you do? You raid the cookie container, eat a candy bar, or down a sugary piece of cake, which compounds vitamin B-1 deficiency and accentuates your irritability, blues, or depression, making you want more junk food fortification. I know. As chapter 1 told you, I've been there—along with Sara Lee.

Totally deprived of vitamin B-1, test subjects in a psychiatric ward exhibited flaring tempers, nervousness, irritability, depression, and frustration. They quarreled and even smashed furniture. When supplied a small amount of vitamin B-1, their attitudes and their conduct improved in every respect.

Vitamin B-6 is another neglected member of the B family. It is easy to avoid in the typical American diet, much to the detriment of your physical and emotional life. Vitamin B-6 is designed into

whole grains, liver, lean muscle meats, fish, nuts (filberts, peanuts, walnuts), sunflower seeds, wheat germ, and bananas, which
are richer by far in this vitamin than any other fruit. The need
for vitamin B-6 grows greater as we age, and some authorities
feel we should supplement what we derive from foods throughout
our lifetime.

Irritability, nervousness, and depression are common signs
of a B-6 deficiency—emotional conditions driving you to eat foods
that you don't always need but that never forget to leave a gen-
erous deposit in your various fat banks.

Niacin is the fourth member of the B family likely to be short
in the typical diet and one that, if not amply supplied, can bring
on nervous disorders, sleeplessness, irritability, and deep depression. Sleeplessness often encourages multiple visits to the refrigerator. The best food sources of niacin are fish, lean meats, poultry,
and peanuts, as well as the food supplements brewer's yeast,
wheat germ, and desiccated liver.

Deficiency of both vitamins B-12 and B-1 often causes irritability (frequently accompanied by depression), slow thinking,
and memory lapses, as demonstrated in numerous starvation experiments. On the other hand, supplying starving subjects with
the missing B-complex vitamins—heavy on the B-1 and B-12—
reduces then eliminates their irritability and depression and improves their thinking and remembering.

An article by Dr. J. MacDonald Holmes in the *British Medical
Journal*, reviewed a number of experiments with vitamin B-12 and
disclosed that an acute deficiency of this vitamin encourages overpowering emotional and mental symptoms: agitated depression,
delusions, visual and auditory hallucinations, maniacal behavior,
and even epilepsy. However, correction of these nutritional shortages brings quick improvement.

In his fine book, *Dr. Wright's Book of Nutritional Therapy*, Jon-
athan Wright, M.D., of Kent, Washington, cites the richest food
sources of vitamin B-12: liver, kidney, muscle meats, fish, and
dairy products. He mentions that in his practice vitamin B-12 plays
a major role in controlling everything from asthma to shingles.
The B-12 resists absorption into the gastrointestinal tract when an
enzyme called the "intrinsic factor" is missing.

Now vitamin makers have added the intrinsic factor to vitamin B-12, and another version of this nutrient is absorbed into the blood stream by melting under the tongue.

Out of the realm of vitamins is a little considered cause of depression, anxiety, and nervousness: low thyroid function. As Stephen Langer, M.D. and James F. Scheer state in their book, *Solved: The Riddle of Illness*: "Depressed persons are more likely to get relief from thyroid supplementation than from warmed over psychotherapy."

Langer says that first-generation hypothyroids often can correct this condition with iodine-rich kelp, the major food for the thyroid gland. However, if they are second-generation hypothyroids or beyond that, they can compensate for their lack only with thyroid hormones prescribed by medical doctors. Langer has achieved the best results with natural thyroid, the kind obtained from animals rather than the synthetic variety.

Thyroid insufficiency is a root cause of much depression and fatigue, as shown by Mark Gold, M.D., and associates at Fair Oaks Hospital in Summit, New Jersey. After examining 350 in-patients and 44 outpatients diagnosed as depressed, Dr. Gold was surprised to find a "significant incidence of low-level hypothyroidism," showing him that depression is often the first manifestation of low-level thyroid failure. This subtle stage of deterioration is not always detected by conventional thyroid function tests.

Only 10 percent of the depressed patients established as hypothyroid had been so diagnosed. Yet, 90 percent of the depressed who showed marked signs of hypothyroidism came out as normal in this category in the usual blood tests.

Untreated subtle hypothyroidism becomes increasingly severe in a short period, Gold soon found. Reduction of depression results from early diagnosis and treatment. Gold stresses that it is imperative to give all psychiatric patients an evaluation for hypothyroidism, because with a reduction of 10 percent in thyroid function, brain function also declines by the same amount. Although a patient with a sluggish thyroid may appear to be normal, he or she will undergo brain changes.

Gold is not surprised that hypothyroids seem to be psychiatric patients who manifest depression. He estimated that 10 percent of the depressed patients who visit psychiatrists have asymptomatic autoimmune thyroiditis, a disorder characterized by the immune system attacking the thyroid gland, causing inflammation and consequent reduced function.

Recently researchers have discovered that though a supposedly symptomless ailment, asymptomatic autoimmune thyroiditis indeed has symptoms, a major one of which is depression. However, Gold has found that most cases of depression are brought on by simple hypothyroidism.

Over and above thyroid supplementation to dissipate depression, many preventive medicine specialists have discovered that various nutrients, especially the amino acid tryptophan, often banish depression nearly miraculously.

A convincing experiment had some patients taking 6 grams a day of tryptophan. They showed significant improvement without side effects. Other patients, taking imipramine, a drug, improved faster but suffered unpleasant and undesirable side effects. The richest natural sources of tryptophan are soybeans, nuts, tuna, and turkey.

Sometimes the trace mineral lithium is used to treat depression. Unfortunately, its reputation for effectiveness and harmlessness is unwarranted. A study by P.L. Rabin and D.C. Evans of the Vanderbilt University School of Medicine demonstrated that lithium worsens depression because it interferes with thyroid function. In an article in the *Journal of Clinical Psychiatry*, Rabin and Evans say, ". . . goiter formation and hypothyroidism are not infrequent following lithium therapy . . ."

Particularly depressing to the obese and heavyweights is the fact that they don't often eat large amounts of food unless they are in an aroused emotional state. However, such emotional arousals can usually be controlled by manipulating environmental conditions and events. Put in specific situational terms, this means that if you are emotionally upset, just detour around the supermarket bakery case displaying those wicked chocolate eclairs.

And while you're still being influenced by negative emotions, don't get involved with three kinds of deprivation that researchers Stuart and Davis have found could undermine your weight control diet: 1) skipping meals 2) neglecting sleep (energy deprivation) and 3) depriving yourself of stimulation (letting yourself become bored).

The danger of skipping meals is that you feel that you owe

it to yourself to overeat at the next meal. Poor sleep (and resulting fatigue) and boredom make you want to overcompensate by over-eating.

Various researchers have discovered that normal-weight people eat because they're hungry whereas the obese eat as a result of various emotional states: depression, boredom, anger, excitement, and happiness.

Dr. Albert J. Stunkard, one of the foremost weight loss authorities, points out that excessive eating, which he calls "reactive eating," results in a drastic lessening of physical activity, as in depression or grief. Such a two-headed program—overeating and under-exercising—can ruin any weight loss program.

Emotionally motivated eating is sometimes called "the night eating syndrome," because it is the heaviest food intake at the time of the least physical activity. It occurs to the obese in the dark of night when the day's fatigue and trials bring on the worst depression.

Stunkard and H.B. Wolff have discovered that obese patients metabolize carbohydrates drastically differently when depressed. It is during such periods that they gain the most weight. Dr. Jean Mayer has a rather unique way of characterizing depression-motivated overeating: "From gloom to gluttony."

Once the negative emotions are under control, it is far easier to follow a dietary regimen to lose weight. And there are many such regimens. Unfortunately, most of the most popular diets have ingredients that doom them from succeeding, but it is educational to consider them and learn what not to do.

CHAPTER FOURTEEN

THE PARADE OF DIETS IS OUT OF STEP

*Take heed to yourselves that your heart be not deceived
. . . Deuteronomy 11:16 (KJV)*

*A*S you review the passing parade of diets, you can't believe what you're seeing and want to rain on the parade. Each new regimen tops the previous one in ridiculousness, as many biochemists keep telling me. The following are parodies on some of the latest:

The Great Garbanzo Bean Diet
The Sensational Sugar Cookie Diet
The Wonderful Watercress Diet

In the Great Garbanzo Bean Diet you eat garbanzo beans until you can't look a garbanzo in the face and you don't feel that great.

The Sensational Sugar Cookie Diet is different. You start each meal with a sugar cookie to trick your mind into thinking it's already dessert time and the meal is over, so you don't eat as much. It works at first, but gradually you begin to eat as much as ever because you are shortchanging your body of needed nutrients and you miss the omitted foods. Now, however, the three sugar cookies a day add several hundred more calories to your usual diet—calories your unkind bathroom scale refuses to ignore.

The Wonderful Watercress Diet will also help initially. Yet how long can you stuff on watercress? By the time chlorophyll

126

starts coming out of your ears, you begin to binge on foods you like.

All the major weight control diets fail because they ignore our connectedness with God through nature. They are man's one-sided, distorted, out-of-balance biochemical caricatures of the way we should really eat. It is virtually impossible for anyone to stay on these diets for two towering reasons. They ignore taste preferences and they ignore nutritional needs, says Adam Drenowski, a University of Michigan nutrition authority.

Examples: the superhigh protein, the superhigh complex carbohydrate, and the superhigh fat diets. Each one is so heavy on a single category of food that it is a distortion of the way we are used to eating. And they all fail to satisfy our requirements for vitamins and minerals.

The following major diets will be reviewed in light of my own experience and inputs from many biochemists and physicians: the Atkins Superenergy Weight Reducing Diet; the Beverly Hills Diet; The Cambridge Plan; The Eat to Win Diet; The F-Plan Diet; Fit for Life; The Grapefruit Diet; The Immune Power Diet; The Pritikin Diet; The Rotation Diet; and The Zen (Macrobiotic) Diet.

Atkins Superenergy Diet

Dr. Atkins doesn't run with the high-carbohydrate lemmings because numerous individuals are intolerant to carbs and have sugar metabolism disorders that contribute to weight gain. No argument from me and my review board.

It is difficult to break down his carbohydrate-protein-fat ratio. However, the diet leans quite heavily on protein, which is slighted in many other diets. It's great to have a high complex carbohydrate diet for energy, but tissue needs to be repaired and rebuilt, and that calls for superior protein.

Dr. Atkins' diet accents reducing carbohydrates—particularly the refined variety—rather than severely slashing calories. I could live with this diet, and friends who have tried it feel the same and have lost weight on it.

The Beverly Hills Diet

After trying this diet, I found myself wishing I had abandoned it in Beverly Hills. This regimen accents conscious food combining, a la Dr. Herbert Shelton. This is a theory never substantiated to anyone's satisfaction but Dr. Shelton, his small coterie, the writer of the Beverly Hills diet, and the Fit for Life people.

You are supposed to eat only certain food groups at one sitting because you weren't born with the enzymes to handle all the food groups in your stomach at one time. Although you came into this world "fearfully and wonderfully made," as it says in Psalms 139:14, God didn't equip you with proper digestion because He hadn't had the foresight to read the Beverly Hills Diet.

Obviously, when your mother was ready to give birth to you, you should have come squawling into the world attached to a "how-to" food-combining manual.

As it turns out, you don't really do much combining in the Beverly Hills diet. You eat a single fruit, such as bananas, all day. Of course, you could combine several bananas in a blender. For eighteen days, you eat a fruit of the day. Then you treat yourself to lobster or steak.

If you thrive on protein starvation, this is the diet for you. Illogical and unbalanced, it shatters many rules of good nutrition and also promotes fluid loss, causing depletion of minerals, including potassium. Among the goodies that often come with the diet are diarrhea, depression, fatigue, and irregular heartbeat.

One day the diet is bananas; the next, it's papayas; and the next, it's mangoes. It all seems monotonous and sickeningly sweet—which it is—but there's something worse. The diet's inordinate amount of fructose (fruit sugar) seems ominous in light of a discovery made by the USDA's Research Section.

Copper deficiency is widely prevalent in the United States due to the eating of so many processed, incomplete, and foodless foods. Intake of excessive fructose, combined with copper deficiency, can cause serious heart damage. Biochemists in the Department of Agriculture's Beltsville, Maryland, research center gave pigs a high-fructose–low-copper diet and found that their hearts doubled in size over that of control group animals.

Mercifully, I couldn't stay on this fruit-heavy regimen long enough to reach Day 18 and liberation. This is what probably saves others from heart damage, too. With this day-after-day routine of sweet, sweet fruits—bananas, pineapple, papaya, mangoes, and watermelon—I must confess, I nearly went bananas.

The Cambridge Plan

This diet features a food powder that comes in many tasty flavors, among them alluring chocolate—one of those nutritional "no-nos" that I wish were a "yes-yes."

Offering only 330 calories a day and a mere 33 grams of protein, the Cambridge Plan seemed unnecessarily restrictive to me. It was far too little for the size appetite I bring to a table. Sure, the protein is high quality from milk and soybeans, but 33 grams a day? Really? The RDA is 44 grams for women and 56 grams for men.

It is no easy matter to stay on this diet, which, to me, is unnecessarily Spartan. My problem with it? I'm no Spartan.

The Eat To Win Diet

An assortment of complex carbohydrates—the performance foods—is the heart of the "Eat To Win" diet. The premise of this regimen is that both protein and fat diminish athletic performance, and the accent is on fresh complex carbohydrates.

Great!

High carbohydrates, low protein, and low fat—in a ratio of approximately 80:12:8—will help you lose weight and improve competitive athletic performance. However, the protein intake for rebuilding tissue is a bit low. Unless more protein is added, you are building up for a letdown.

One of the diet's artificial aspects is a dietary regimen for different sports. Hey, fella, energy output is energy output. Of course, these different diets that slim you down help to fatten up the book.

As an aerobic dancer, scuba diver, tennis buff, and skier, I found that the diet boosted my performance initially, but that in time I began to lose energy without understanding why. Luke Bucci, Ph.D., my biochemist friend, advised me to take free-form amino acids on the side. He also mentioned something that most sports diets—most diets, for that matter—miss for individuals who go in for heavy exertion activities such as distance running: a common disorder for athletes these days known as "sports anemia."

As Luke explains it, "Strenuous exercise burns up iron fast. Most people who are into athletics don't usually eat enough of the proper foods to resupply themselves with iron. They are often strict or modified vegetarians.

"Vigorous activity boosts body temperature, revs up blood circulation, and changes blood chemistry, using up iron-rich blood hemoglobin rapidly. This is where a good protein such as meat is needed to supply iron.

"We all remember Popeye draining a can of spinach to develop superhuman energy. Spinach is loaded with iron, but it contains oxalic acid which combines with vitally needed calcium and carries it out of the body.

"Taking them alphabetically, the best foods for iron content are blackstrap molasses, brown rice, chickpeas, dried apricot, meat, lima beans, liver, oysters, poultry (particularly duck), pistachio nuts, raisins, walnuts, wheat bran, and white beans."

"And, of course," he concludes, "iron is best absorbed when taken with vitamin C-rich foods like oranges or orange juice or the vitamin C supplement itself—usually no less than 500 milligrams a day."

Luke proved to be right. Free-form amino acids and iron brought me back. However, the Eat to Win Diet gave me an uncomfortably full feeling in the stomach, and friends of mine experienced similar feelings along with diarrhea.

With my decline of energy and pep on this particular regimen, I have to say that the Eat to Win Diet threw me for a loss.

The F-Plan Diet

Increase the bulk in your diet—that is, add 35 to 50 grams of high-fiber foods daily—and thus reduce your intake and calories. That's the principle of the F-Plan Diet.

Many fibers are water-retentive to give you a feeling of full-ness, and you tend to slosh around all day. But the principle is good. In addition to all the fiber, you get to eat two pieces of whole fresh fruit, and you get to drink some fruit juices and 8 ounces of skim milk.

One objection to the diet is that a heavy fiber intake in some individuals hurries food through so fast it hasn't enough time to leave off its nutrients.

Initially, I felt inflation setting in and an uncomfortably full feeling, but that's the general idea. I give the F-Plan an "F" grade—not for failure but for fine.

Fit For Life

In this retread of the Beverly Hills Diet and Shelton Natural Hygiene, we again have food combining and enough fruit to make you go ape.

As a matter of fact, I ate so much fruit on this diet that I may not touch it again for the rest of my life. Everyone I know who has tried this diet—with one exception—was unable to stay on it.

The Fit for Life regimen violates the way human beings eat, fails to supply sufficient nutrients (especially protein) and, as with the high fructose intake in the Beverly Hills Diet, poses the threat of heart damage in individuals who are copper-deficient.

The diet and the book on which it is based are filled with specious premises, such as that eggs are not good for you, not only because they contain fat and cholesterol but because they have all that smelly sulfur. Why then did God make the human body with a content of 2.5 percent sulfur?

I know the authors, and they are wonderfully creative peo-ple. Their second book, *Living Health,* is supremely enjoyable read-ing.

During the time I was able to hang in there on the Fit For Life diet, I experienced every diabolical digestive disturbance be-cause I am a Candida sufferer. Candida, a yeast overgrowth in the intestines and elsewhere in the body, can cause illness or, in extreme cases, death. Individuals with Candida albicans must go easy on the intake of sugars, even from fruit. A friend suggested that if I stayed with the Fit For Life diet, I would begin to like it and lose weight, too, even if I had nothing to lose.

"No, thanks," I replied. "I would rather be fat for life."

The Grapefruit Diet

Weight reduction experts at Michael Reese Hospital in Chicago feel that the grapefruit, as a melter of excess poundage, is an imposter.

"The premise is that grapefruit has an enzyme that breaks down faster, so that you can eat a lot, and the grapefruit will keep you slim," says Murray J. Favus, M.D. "Well, the body breaks down enzymes on their way to the stomach. If grapefruit does have such an enzyme, it's destroyed before it can do anything."

The Immune Power Diet

The book, *Dr. Berger's Immune Power Diet* makes solid sense. What is something so sensible doing amid so much nonsense? Its theme is that food sensitivities and allergies can make one gain or retain weight, so let's identify and eliminate them. Also, the valid point is made that an immune system constantly busy fighting off allergens and partially digested foods in the bloodstream doesn't have much left to defend against real enemies.

People I know who have tried this diet have lost weight and something else worth losing—a swarm of allergy-produced symptoms: eye watering, itches, sneezes, sniffles, and wheezes.

The Pritikin Permanent Weight Loss Diet

All the raw vegetables you can eat make this a great diet if you are a vegetarian. The Pritikin diet is top-heavy in complex carbohydrates. However, in this version of it, more protein has been added—up to RDA level.

That's progress. Nevertheless, there should be a built-in margin to compensate for protein lost under stress. And many of us do not handle stress properly. Although the diet permits egg whites, it does not allow egg yolks and omits lecithin, which is a must for a healthy liver.

The Pritikin phobia of saturated fats is manifest in this diet, which is roughly 80 percent complex carbohydrates, 12 percent protein, and 8 percent fat. It is true that the American diet is overloaded with fats—over 40 percent—and a 10 percent cut is endorsed by diet experts across the board. But going down to 8 percent may present health problems we can't even imagine.

However, there is some merit in this plan.

The Rotation Diet

Slash your calories to a minimum and exercise moderately, and you are supposed to lose on the Rotation Diet. Who can quarrel with this premise?

There is a small problem with the Rotation Diet. Who can stay on it? You supposedly keep your metabolism in high gear by rotating from an extremely low-cal week—between 600 and 900 calories—to a week of medium-cal days—around 1200 calories. The variation in caloric intake is supposed to keep metabolism high.

Although the carbohydrate-to protein-to fat ratio is reasonable—50:25:25—there are many nutrient deficiencies in the diet. Meat, poultry, fish, and dairy products are included. Hooray. However, the diet is somewhat boring. I found myself rebelling against it.

Besides all other liquids, you are required to drink 64 ounces of water daily. Sometimes you feel as if you're carrying around a small swimming pool.

So far as the Rotation Diet is concerned, I found myself wishing I could get rotated right out of it. I could and did.

The Zen (Macrobiotic) Diet

The premise of this diet always reminds me of the story of the man who kept feeding his plow horse less and less each day and tried to get the same amount of work out of him. For a while the plan seemed all right, but one morning the man found the horse collapsed on the straw of the stall, never again to eat or work.

This macrobiotic diet requires progressively more food restriction until you are reduced to nothing but brown rice and herb tea. Being accustomed to eating varied foods, I felt like screaming as I endured this daily discipline.

Dr. Lynne Levitsky of Michael Reese Hospital in Chicago characterizes the macrobiotic diet better than I can:

"It's a disaster nutritionally, and the insidious thing about it is that the rice fills you up, so you may be starving but not feel hungry!"

Richard B. Friedman, M.D., vice chairman of the Department of Medicine and director of the Weight Reduction Program at the University of Wisconsin, Madison, says that a regimen as extreme as the macrobiotic diet is nutritionally unsound, "self-imposed starvation," and extremely dangerous.

You can certainly lose weight on it. You can also certainly die on it, as some individuals have. I finally abandoned the macrobiotic diet. After all, I'm not dying to lose weight!

Dr. Friedman made a survey of all types of diets—from fad diets to sound ones with every calorie level involved. He discovered many, if not most, individuals lose weight if they take in less than 1500 calories daily. Some test subjects, even with normal thyroid function, have to reduce calories sharply—to 1000 calories daily—to continue shedding unwanted weight.

The best and most effective diets bring about slow and often frustrating results: roughly a half pound a week. Yet these are the most sound. You didn't gain your weight all at once, and you should lose it in much the same way—gradually. It is a sad commentary that people who endure the 1000-calorie-a-day regimen to lose all of their excess weight, usually regain it within a year or two by going back to their old eating patterns.

Dr. Friedman maintains that, in the beginning, every diet brings about weight loss because it slashes calories below the body's requirements. However, as shown in my review of the major diets, many are too restrictive and boring, making it a chore to adhere to them. Then, too, some diets are health hazards.

Most effective weight loss diets are about 50 percent carbo-hydrates, 15 to 20 percent protein, and 30 to 35 percent fat. The percentage of fat is a reasonable decline from the estimated 40 to 45 percent of the present American diet. We can live with that more easily than with the sharp reduction of fat in most diets.

Dr. Friedman strongly advises dieters to play it safe, taking in the recommended daily allowances of major food classifica-tions, protein, vitamins, and minerals within the calorie range of 1000 to 1800 daily according to their weight.

Rather than critique the major diets—fad or sound—by name, Dr. Friedman rates them according to their substance, or lack of it.

Setpoint

Lowering your setpoint to lose weight is neither novel nor proved, states Dr. Friedman. It is an old concept with a new name. You simply lower your caloric intake to 1200 to 1800 daily and exercise moderately. This program, even in animal experiments, has not been proved by adequate testing. (Some authorities dis-agree with Dr. Friedman. See chapter 11 for a detailed discussion of setpoint.)

High-Carbohydrate

Complex carbohydrates with their high fluid content—fruits and vegetables—increase bulk and make you feel fine. Such a diet, added to exercise and behavior modification, has merit.

High-Fiber

Low in both calories and protein, the high-fiber diet—35 to 50 grams a day—is considered to bind fat and protein and thus give the feeling of satiation. Dr. Friedman feels that all claims (some of them extravagant) are not documented well enough, but he is convinced that added fiber improves the diet.

══════════════ *Low-Carbohydrate* ══════════════

It is almost a truism that low-carbohydrate diets are also low in fats. Insufficient carbohydrates to oxidize fats cause a medical condition known as ketosis with symptoms of dehydration, diarrhea, sodium depletion, excess blood fats, exhaustion, and postural hypertension.

══════════════ *High-Protein* ══════════════

Although you can be a good weight loser on this one, Dr. Friedman feels the regimen is monotonous and therefore hard to stay on over a long period. Usually high in cholesterol and fats, the high-protein diet is not well handled by individuals plagued with diabetes, gout, or kidney or liver disease, or by pregnant women.

Copious amounts of water should be taken with it, so that the body can rid itself of ketones, the harmful chemicals resulting from the body's attempt to burn fats for energy with little or no carbohydrates present to help. Excessive ketones bring on bad breath and fatigue.

══════════════ *High-Fat* ══════════════

This is the best tasting diet. It moves slowly through the digestive tract and therefore gives eaters a feeling of satiation for a longer time. Of course, warns Friedman, it is hazardous to the health of individuals with hypercholesterolemia, but this is a small percentage of the population.

However, as explained in chapter 7, "Go Easy on Fat Foods," dietary fat has a way of becoming body fat more readily than do proteins and carbohydrates—a fact that is part of today's sometimes clarifying, sometimes confusing, information explosion on diet, health, and fitness.

DON'T LET WEIGHT LOSS MYTHS UNDERMINE YOU

My people are destroyed for lack of knowledge. Hosea 4:6 (KJV)

*D*ISTINGUISHING fact from fiction about weight loss is like trying to separate strands of cooked spaghetti. It can be done, but it's difficult. If you don't know myth from reality, you may not lose weight and could even gain some. Horrors! Remember, a myth is as good as a mile.

Should you fail to know the correct answers for even half of the following true or false statements, you may be your own greatest impediment to winning the losing game.

1. *One of the best ways to lose weight is to skip meals, particularly breakfast.* **FALSE.** Meal skipping is one of the worst ways devised by man to lose weight, particularly because most individuals skip the day's meals most crucial to health—breakfast and lunch. If you decide upon this form of self-torture, skip dinner.

When I checked on the findings of several preventive medicine specialists, I learned that most of their patients gain weight on meal skipping. When they omit breakfast or lunch, they experience the rebound effect: overcompensating by eating extra calories in the two meals that follow. A small breakfast—donuts and coffee or toast and juice—produces almost as much late-morning inefficiency and fatigue as skipping breakfast. A breakfast including eggs and milk keeps the blood sugar level high until lunch. Lesser breakfasts don't.

In investigating 1000 accidents in ordnance depots, Army efficiency engineers discovered that most of the injured workers had reported to work without having eaten breakfast. Fatigue and carelessness due to low blood sugar led to their having accidents.

Seventy-five percent of all industrial accidents occur to people who have not eaten breakfast. Over and above carelessness, we become irritable, exhausted, and ravenously hungry, subconsciously determined to compensate at lunch and dinner for our martyrdom in skipping breakfast.

A survey of 50,000 students of all ages revealed that 16 percent—8000—ate no breakfast at all and that almost 65 percent ate breakfasts that were inadequate for the physical requirements. This may be one reason why American students are also-rans in world academic ratings.

Several researchers have learned that it is important to eat the heaviest meals nearest the time of greatest energy expenditure. The American habit of eating the biggest and highest fat content meal at night when we need it the least—to fuel us with energy to watch TV or to sleep—is tailor-made to add unwanted weight.

Breakfast is the day's most important meal because it gives us the charge we need to get through all of our activities. A study by the U.S. Department of Agriculture revealed that breakfast eaters—eaters of an egg, a slice of whole grain toast, and a glass of orange juice—sustain a high blood sugar level (one of the major determinants of high energy) compared with those who have only a cup of coffee or a cup of coffee and a donut.

As a matter of fact, the full-breakfast eaters sustain a higher blood sugar level even after lunch than do the coffee and the coffee-and-donut groups.

You steal from your own mental alertness and efficiency if you skip breakfast. This is a finding of a ten-year study directed by two State University of Iowa investigators, Dr. W.W. Tuttle, professor of physiology, and Dr. Kate Daum, director of nutrition at the university hospitals.

During the first phase of the research, half of the study's fifty subjects—whose ages ranged from 12 to 83—ate a morning meal as well as lunch and dinner. The other half had the same menu but ate only at lunch and dinnertime. After two to four weeks, the test subjects swapped schedules.

The researchers found that breakfast skippers of all age groups showed a sharp decline of physical and mental efficiency, and that those who failed to eat breakfast did not lose weight.

Many of my viewers have written, "I'm not hungry and can't eat breakfast."

Yes, you can! Just skip dinner for several nights, and you'll begin to get back into a normal and effective eating pattern. That's the only meal it's safe to omit.

2. *If you eat more than three times a day but still stay within your reduced calorie limit, you won't upset your weight reduction diet.* **TRUE.** As a matter of fact, many human and animal studies have disclosed that five to seven small meals of the same caloric value as three meals will usually produce greater weight loss.

Dr. Paul Lynn of San Francisco asked fifty-three overweight patients to eat many small meals daily. He achieved a startling success rate. About 80 percent of them dropped a half pound to a pound a week, whereas on an equal number of calories consumed in three meals, they had been gaining a quarter to a half a pound a week.

This finding is especially encouraging in that these patients did nothing additional to shed excess weight. They didn't even exercise. One of the prime benefits of this plan is that numerous small meals give you a feeling of satiation, keep your blood sugar elevated to offer you sufficient energy, and fend off binge-promoting emotional negatives such as anxiety, feelings of insecurity, and depression.

Are there benefits other than gradual weight loss to the frequent feeding method? On the basis of animal studies—Biochemist Richard Passwater states that many small meals are easy on our complicated digestion and food transport system. Further, they do not stress the reserves of various organs, including the heart.

3. *The meal reversal pattern is effective in encouraging weight loss or control—that is, eating the heaviest meal in the morning,* *a lighter one at noon, and the lightest at night.* **TRUE!** A meal reversal experiment with 595 overweight individuals in reasonably good health was reported in the *Journal of the Louisiana State Medical Society*. These test subjects were asked to change a lifetime's eating habits while eating the same number of daily calories they usually consumed.

Participants lost five to six pounds monthly on average. Those who stayed with the program and dropped twenty to thirty pounds were found to have an increased blood hemoglobin level. Diabetics who melted off thirty or more pounds returned to normal blood sugar. Likewise, hypothyroids who dropped thirty pounds were able to get along on less thyroid gland supplementation.

4. *Eating a whole grapefruit benefits you by burning up excess fat.* **FALSE.** In chapter 14, "The Parade of Diets Is Out of Step," an authority on weight loss blasts this widely prevalent notion. Supposedly an enzyme exists in grapefruit that dissolves fat. Yet, says this expert, if such an enzyme exists, it gets lost in the stomach's digestive juices. A great fruit to include at breakfast, the grapefruit is impotent so far as a weight loss program is concerned.

5. *Yogurt, called* **laban** *in Bible times, can be considered a meal in itself for a dietary program.* **FALSE.** Yogurt is an excellent food, but it is a form of milk—fermented and easier to take by some milk-intolerants. Experiments by Dr. Joseph Kolars at the University of Minnesota revealed that some 80 percent of those who could not drink milk without all the rumblings of an intestinal civil war were able to tolerate yogurt.

Beware of flavored yogurt, which often contains sugar and adds anywhere from 60 to 120 extra calories to an 8-ounce container. Better to slice up a small piece of fresh fruit into yogurt if you need a sweetener.

6. *Meat and whole milk contain no more cholesterol than fish.* **TRUE.** Despite current propaganda, new evidence reveals that many meat fats have no effect on blood cholesterol, according to Edward R. Pinckney, M.D., and Cathey Pinckney in *The Cholesterol Controversy*.

Many individuals don't eat meat because they feel that using fish and poultry in its place will save their hearts and promote longevity. However, there are adequate studies demonstrating that beef and other meats "contain no more cholesterol than fish fillets."

7. *An all fruit and vegetable diet is nutritionally sound and one of the best regimens for losing weight.* FALSE. Despite information in many best-selling books to this effect, fruits and vegetables are deficient in protein. As chapter 5, "Imitation Foods for Real People," states, protein content of grains and other plant products is steadily declining because present commercial fertilizers do not return to the soil what is taken out by the crops.

Further, fruits and vegetables are usually deficient in vitamin B-12, the lack of which can contribute to pernicious anemia, a devastating disorder. Although it is true that this sort of diet will contribute mightily to weight loss or weight control, it is difficult for many non–fruitarian-vegetarians to adhere to this kind of regimen. Another deficiency in fruits and vegetables in most states is zinc.

8. *Foods must be properly combined. Miscombined foods putrefy in the digestive tract.* FALSE. Such a theory is believed by a small handful of groups and individuals, but it lacks scientific substantiation. In chapter 14, "The Parade of Diets Is Out of Step," I mention that the principle of food combining almost makes it seem that God should have consulted with the writers of two best-selling weight loss books to have equipped us better with enzymes and digestive juices to handle all types of food at once.

In *The University of California, Berkeley Wellness Letter*, Dr. Sheldon Margen, professor of public health nutrition, claims that there is a lack of scientific evidence backing food combining. Advocates of food combining claim that unlike foods, such as proteins and starches, fat and starches, and proteins and sugar, should not be eaten at the same meal. These incompatibles require different digestive juices (enzymes) and processes. Thus miscombinations putrefy in the intestinal tract, producing poisons that "paralyze the intestines," block elimination of waste, and spill toxins into the bloodstream. Properly combined foods supposedly detoxify the body.

Margen says that these strictures would rule out nearly every common dish: macaroni and cheese, meat and cheese sandwiches, and most Mexican entrees. People who advocate food combining rarely deal with the issue that all foods—even those eaten individually—contain combinations of carbohydrates, fat, and protein. Whole milk is made up of almost equal amounts of these food categories.

Foods rich in vitamin C help the body absorb iron in grains. Yet food combiners would not tolerate such a combination. Another sensible point is the fact that vitamins and minerals are more efficiently used when eaten as a part of a conglomerate of foods instead of as part of a single substance.

Margen points out that when a calcium pill is taken with a manganese pill (both are essential to bone building), the calcium impedes absorption of the manganese. Yet when the calcium of milk meets with manganese, the two are compatible.

Healthy individuals digest and absorb something like 98 percent of carbohydrates, fats, and proteins with efficiency—an excellent inside job without help from the outside.

9. *A cup of orange juice is lower in calories and more advantageous for dieting than a medium-size orange, and nut butter is lower in calories than an equivalent weight of nuts.* **FALSE.** A whole orange is more satisfying than a glass of orange juice because it has more bulk and takes longer to eat. It also contains thirty-five fewer calories. Also, nut butters are more concentrated and calorie-packed than the nuts from which they are made.

10. *Low thyroid function contributes to the inability of many individuals to lose weight.* **TRUE.** Proper working of the thyroid gland keeps various body systems operating properly. In the hypothyroid (an individual with low thyroid function) food cannot be efficiently broken down and absorbed through the gastrointestinal mucosa. Assimilation is often faulty in the hypothyroid, and the heartbeat is not usually strong enough to transport food and oxygen to the farthest-out cells. Wastes must also be efficiently eliminated from cells and transported by the circulatory system to the liver and kidneys for detoxification and discharged through bowels, bladder, skin, and lungs. All of these processes are moderate to weak in the hypothyroid.

Decreased oxygen use and lowered rate of heat production mean a decrease in metabolism and an inability to lose weight. When the bathroom scale spitefully refuses to move lower, the body has set its thermostat lower due to worsening hypothyroidism.

Despite all that has gone before, hypothyroidism doesn't always make you retain weight, says thyroid expert Dr. Broda Barnes, indicating that more than 40 percent of his tens of thousands of hypothyroid patients in a long career were actually underweight. He advises, however, that if you are both overweight and hypothyroid, you may need to take thyroid hormone to make your weight control diet work.

11. *Long-stored fat—an unwelcome guest for months or years—is harder to burn off than newly acquired fat.* **TRUE.** New fat has not as yet had a chance to entrench itself. Experts on body fat say that membranes of old fat cells are more resistant than those of newer fat cells. Therefore, it is harder to burn off the fat in older fat cells.

12. *It is possible to keep weight off permanently on many diets.* **TRUE.** However, most individuals will not or cannot do what needs to be done to make these diets work. The secret is to follow a modified diet for life—not just for several weeks. (One problem is that many diets are nutrient-poor and could be harmful if followed permanently.)

A high price tag is often attached to protracted and steady dieting: exhaustion, depression, illness from malnourishment, and living only a fractional life, with all of which come frequent long, deep sighs and the feeling of "what's the use?"

Few people can modify their usual eating habits after the dieting is over. School is out. Responding to intense and gnawing hunger, they eat just about the way they did before. Authorities say that if the diet resulted in a ten- to fifteen-pound loss in the first couple of weeks, most people will regain all the lost weight within about two months after the death of the diet.

13. *When on a weight loss diet, it is not a good idea to drink a great deal of water (eight to ten glasses daily) because this much fluid only contributes to undesired water retention.* **FALSE.** Drinking so much water produces just the opposite effect. It fights fluid retention, signaling the body that it can release stored fluids. Consuming a lot of water has two additional benefits: fluid contributes to the metabolizing of fat, and it restrains appetite.

14. *Diet drinks can make you put on weight!* **TRUE!** How can that be? They're supposed to be diet drinks, right? Dr. Dennis Remington, director of the Eating Disorder Clinic at Brigham Young University, states that artificial sweeteners, hundreds of times sweeter than sugar, develop a craving in individuals for sweets that makes many of them reach for a cookie, sweet roll, or candy bar. Thus diet drinks work in the opposite way than intended.

The diet drink fools the taste buds, making them react as they would to real sugar. So the body, expecting an intake of more sugar, may release additional insulin, which could lead to weight gain.

15. *You can keep your arteries young by means of regular, vigorous physical workouts through aerobic weight loss exercises.* **TRUE.** The smooth muscle fibers that line the blood vessels must be exercised or they tend to lose their flexibility and harden. How do you do this? You walk briskly for more than thirty minutes, or jog, run, or cycle, so that your heart pumps harder and faster, sending a pulsating stream of blood carrying oxygen and nutrients throughout your body.

With each contraction followed by an expansion of your heart, the blood makes the blood vessels expand and contract, really exercising them. Little used blood vessels become flabby and eventually more susceptible to medical disorders and then more susceptible to degenerative changes such as inflexibility and hardening. This is why physical activity should be part of everyday's regimen—a way of life.

16. *There's no foolproof way to test and tell if various forms of aerobic exercise are beyond your physical condition.* **FALSE.** Your body has a built-in warning system: being overtired, out of breath, or becoming dizzy. Before risking these symptoms, you should have a complete physical exam and get a clearance from your doctor.

Then, start a slow-paced walk until normally tired. The symptoms listed above will tell you when you're exceeding your present physical capacities. Each day you can exercise a little more vigorously and longer before the warning signs appear. Wholesome, spirited exercise should not cause pain—during or after it is performed.

17. *All vigorous aerobic weight loss exercises performed on foot invariably damage knees or ankles.* **FALSE.** Jogging, running, and dancing may cause harm to these parts of the legs, but fast walking will not. Even jogging and running can be performed without danger of injury if these physical activities are practiced on a running track or on level, smooth grass—or even on hard surfaces provided the athletic shoes worn have soles with give to them.

When a jogger's foot hits the ground, the impact value is three times greater than his body weight. The ankles and knees of a 150-pounder take a 450-pound jolt with each footfall. Aerobic dancers take an even harder impact—four times their body weight.

Do these findings suggest we give up exercising to protect ankles and knees? No, only that we take all necessary precautions: finding running surfaces that are moderately soft so that impacts are reduced, or wearing cushioned shoes for the very same reason.

18. *Obesity is not desirable and should always be dealt with.* **FALSE.** In most instances, obesity brings on various physical disorders and may lessen the lifespan. However, some individuals live long just by following a regular, aerobic exercise program. Trying to cope with obesity by repeated weight loss regimens followed by weight gains may be self-defeating and harmful to the body. It is best to find a dietary and exercise regimen you can live with and adhere to for the rest of your life.

19. *Bicycling—moving or stationary—is the best aerobic exercise of all for losing weight.* **TRUE.** Dr. Grant Gwinup, who bicycles daily and is greyhound lean, says it burns off even more calories than does running. It is his favorite physical activity.

If you're out of condition, you can start with a few minutes of easy pedaling on a level road. If you become winded or exhausted, you're pushing your body too hard. Ease up. Some authorities recommend a break from arduous riding with several minutes of slower pedaling. Leave record-breaking rides for somebody in better condition than you are.

The following will give you a good idea how many calories you can burn off through cycling. Just for the sake of statistics, let's assume that you weigh about 165 pounds. If you cycle 5.5 miles per hour, you will melt off 285 calories; 9.5 miles per hour will melt 450 calories; and 13.1 miles per hour will melt off 750 calories.

One more advantage of cycling over jogging and running is that you don't beat your ankles and knees to death impacting hard pavement.

20. *If you select clothing that camouflages your overweight, you will be less inclined to continue on a weight loss program.* **FALSE.** Bariatrics experts tell me that people who care enough about their appearance to buy clothing that creates the illusion of a longer and leaner physique also tend to work to slenderize their body.

Meanwhile, while they're psyching themselves up on the inside to make the outside look better, here's what they can do to improve the outside: Stay with one color scheme and let color flow from one piece to the other with no abrupt break. Men's shoes, socks and trousers should match.

To make the body appear taller and more slender, both women and men should avoid horizontal stripes or patterns and huge prints. Women should use shoulder pads and men should wear cuffless pants, which help sell the illusion of height.

Use the magician's technique of drawing the viewer's eyes away from what you don't want seen. Draw attention away from large hips or any other less pleasant feature by drawing the focus to the face with a spectacular hat and earrings. For men straight-legged trousers and vests draw the eyes from the body up to the face.

Loose-fitting, beltless coat dresses are ideal for overweight women, and fullness in the skirt front conceals a bulge that is best hidden. Women with fleshy hips should never wear slim skirts or pants. Skimpy shirts, pants and jackets do nothing but display flab. Men should avoid them.

Simplicity and conservatism are proper for both women's and men's shirts. V-neck collars and open shirts give the illusion of greater thinness.

Know thy bad points, so you can dress to neutralize them. Precise grooming, tidy, pressed, well-fitting, and immaculate clothing will de-emphasize what needs to be de-emphasized. Faddish or trendy clothes tend to accent overweight.

Start liking yourself. Focus on your good points. Let your light within shine.

If you follow these recommendations as you work on a weight reduction plan, there's a good chance that you will soon have a lot less of yourself to like a lot more. However, first it would pay to look into the numerous, little-recognized blockages to losing weight, the subject of the next chapter.

CHAPTER SIXTEEN

HIDDEN CAUSES
OF OVERWEIGHT

Catch us the foxes, the little foxes that spoil the vineyards
. . . Song of Solomon 2:15 (RSV)

*I*N the spirit of the above scripture, be alert to catch the stealthy little foxes that may be nibbling away at your physical and emotional health and in the process frustrating your efforts to lose weight.

Unless you catch the little foxes, they'll keep working you over. So the purpose of this chapter is to help you do just that.

In all honesty, I wasn't fully aware that certain subtle, hard-to-detect ailments often block the most sincere and strenuous efforts to lose weight until I read the book *Solved: The Riddle of Weight Loss*, by two friends, Stephen Langer, M.D., and James F. Scheer.

Langer and Scheer present numerous case studies and valid research projects to substantiate the fact that six little foxes are doing a number on many of us: hypothyroidism (low thyroid function); Candida albicans (a yeast infection); hypoglycemia (low blood sugar); food allergies; stress; and heavy metals intoxication. Then they show how to cope with them and lose weight. By special permission from the authors, I am paraphrasing some information from their book and adding some of my own in these areas.

Let me deal with these little foxes in the order mentioned above:

Hypothyroidism (Low Thyroid Function)

An eminent authority on the thyroid gland, with more than a hundred publications in scientific journals, Broda Barnes has for many years been telling the world that hypothyroidism is the most common disease entering the doctor's office and the diagnosis most often missed. Many times when we addressed National Health Federation conventions from the same platform, I have heard him say, on the basis of some forty-four years of clinical experience, that no less than 40 percent of the United States population is suffering from hidden and undiagnosed low thyroid function.

I remember thinking this a gross exaggeration until I compared notes with Dr. Langer and other northern California preventive medicine specialists, who bore these statistics out by their own findings.

In recent years the Barnes statement has been validated by a rash of articles by authorities such as Gerald S. Levey, an endocrinologist and chief of medicine at the University of Pittsburgh School of Medicine; Leonard J. Kryston, M.D., assistant professor in clinical medicine, University of Pennsylvania; and Mark Gold, M.D., of Fair Oaks Hospital, Summit, New Jersey.

How come all the hidden hypothyroidism?

Glad you asked. Dr. Langer told me that lab tests are "specific for hypothyroidism but not quite sensitive enough." Sadly, many doctors lean hard on the lab tests and almost throw out the patient and his or her symptoms.

Another friend, Edward R. Pinckney, M.D., former associate editor of the *Journal of the American Medical Association*, stands for the old-fashioned way of doctoring using results of laboratory tests in the light of the patient's medical history and symptoms and then making a clinical judgment. "If the doctor doesn't do this, what good are his or her training or experience?" asks Dr. Pinckney.

However, the medical orthodoxy is enamored of lab tests even if they are inaccurate. This is mainly to eliminate malpractice suits, rather than patients.

Dr. Barnes devised a foolproof test for hypothyroidism, a

no-cost temperature test that you can give yourself. Many decades ago, the research that led to the Barnes Basal Temperature Test was reported in the *Journal of the American Medical Association*. The test was also listed in the *Physicians Desk Reference* (PDR) through many annual volumes. Finally, it was dropped, probably because the medical orthodoxy realized that the test cost nothing to the patient. A no-cost test is not worth a cent that it doesn't cost.

What all this melts down to is that you can get a pretty good idea whether or not you are hypothyroid simply by following the Barnes method. Shake down a plain ol' thermometer before going to bed at night and leave it on the nightstand. When you wake up in the morning after a good sleep, stay quiet and place the thermometer in your armpit for ten minutes. Do this for two consecutive days. If your temperature is below the range of 97.8 to 98.2, chances are you are hypothyroid.

Take these results, your symptoms, your medical history, and yourself to a preventive medicine specialist or a wholistic doctor and go from there. If the yellow pages can't direct you to a physician in these categories, get a referral from your nearest health food store.

The major symptoms of hypothyroidism are deep fatigue and cold hands and feet or just being cold all over when most people in the same room are comfortable. Let's run through the other twenty-five most common symptoms:

1. Weight gain or inability to lose weight.
2. Dry, coarse skin.
3. Lethargy.
4. Slow or slurring speech.
5. Constipation.
6 Swelling of face and/or eyelids.
7. Thick tongue.
8. Coarse hair.
9. Diminished ability to sweat (tied into being cold physically).
10. Pale skin.
11. Loss of hair.
12. Labored breathing.

13. Swollen feet.
14. Loss of appetite.
15. Hoarseness.
16. Every menstrual complication—inordinate pain, insufficient or too copious flow, irregular periods or their cessation for the wrong reasons.
17. Nervousness.
18. Heart palpitation.
19. Brittle nails.
20. Slow movement.
21. Slow thinking–poor memory.
22. Depression.
23. Emotional instability.
24. Headaches.
25. High cholesterol level (see chapter 6.).

Because lab tests often show low-thyroid patients as normal, orthodox doctors tend to ignore this laundry list of symptoms. They are unable to diagnose them properly because they don't fit into the orthodox medical box of ready categories, and so they often place these labels on them: 1) "nothing organically wrong," 2) "psychogenic problems," 3) "hypochondriac," or 4) "neurotic."

What is pertinent here is the fact that when the thyroid is underfunctioning, which means that the basal metabolic rate is subnormal, it is difficult to lose weight. Blood circulates sluggishly, nutrients are poorly assimilated, and body wastes are not efficiently eliminated. If low thyroid is not first ruled out, many of this disease's hundred or more symptoms are sadly mistaken for other serious medical conditions and often wrongly treated.

Low-thyroid persons seem to have been born tired, get worse year after year, and become depressed. This sad combination decreases their stamina and makes them poor candidates to sustain a weight loss program. Besides, their low metabolism—the rate at which nutrients are burned for body heat and energy—makes their battle against fat almost impossible to win.

So, if you're hypothyroid, what can you do? Dr. Langer advises adding iodine-containing foods to the diet: saltwater fish—cod, haddock, halibut, and herring. Food supplements such as kelp and cod liver oil contain iodine. If cod liver oil is yucky to you, you might consider capsules, or its mint, cherry, or strawberry flavored versions.

Taking supplemental iodine may help if you are a first-generation hypothyroid. However, if you are a second-generation hypothyroid or even a third, this probably won't work. According to Dr. Langer, if your parents were born in a Goiter Belt area and you were brought up there, you will probably need the thyroid supplement, a prescription item.

Now what and where is a Goiter Belt? A Goiter Belt is an area where iodine has been leached from the soil, where the soil has about one-seventh the iodine needed to be passed on to you by plants and animals.

The world's Goiter Belts are located in mountainous or inland areas—the Alps, Carpathian, and Pyrenees mountain ranges in Europe; the Himalayas of Asia; the Andes mountains of South America; the Appalachian and the Rocky mountains of the United States; the Great Lakes Basin and on west through Minnesota—the Dakotas, Montana, Wyoming (and adjoining regions of Canada); and into the northwest—mainly inland parts of Oregon, Washington, and British Columbia.

An infinitesimal amount of thyroid hormone in each of your cells is like a carburetor. Unless there is enough of it, your biochemical motor won't run efficiently or well—neither will your metabolism. Dr. Langer doesn't mean to convey the impression that every hypothyroid is overweight. In fact, both he and Dr. Barnes discovered that some 39 percent of hypothyroids are normal-weights.

However, there is still that remaining 61 percent. If you are overweight and hypothyroid, see the right doctor, as discussed earlier. If you don't eliminate hypothyroidism, you're fighting great odds. Your Battle of the Bulge could end up being the 100 Years' War.

Candida Albicans (Yeast Infection)

This is a disease that orthodox medicine says doesn't exist—something like hypoglycemia (low blood sugar), which, to traditional medicine, also didn't exist some thirty years ago. Anything that orthodox medicine says doesn't exist, doesn't exist. Perhaps, for the benefit of civilization, this body should ignore AIDS.

Exactly what is Candida albicans? It is an overgrowth (infection) of a form of yeast fungus that has been with us since the beginning of civilization. It thrives in moist warm places of the body: the anus, intestines, nose, throat, and vagina.

A rare medical disorder not many decades ago—it was kept under control in the human anatomy by friendly bacteria—Candida albicans became a serious threat to health, well-being, and even survival with the introduction and widespread use of antibiotics since World War II; high dosages of cortisone; greatly increased consumption of refined carbohydrates in recent years (mainly refined sugar) and increased utilization of the birth control pill.

Antibiotics aimed at harmful bacteria also kill off friendly bacteria, natural defenders that keep Candida under control. Heavy intake of sugar ensures this fungus a rich supply of its favorite food, and heavy use of cortisone and the Pill create ideal conditions for its growth and spread.

Dr. Langer has found that women seem more susceptible to Candida than men by a margin of two and a half to one. And the one major physical characteristic of Candida in young to post-menopausal women, he notes, is the tendency to gain weight—anywhere from fifteen to fifty pounds.

What can be done about this condition? Dr. Langer successfully treats Candida albicans by having patients eliminate sugar and other refined carbohydrates and ingest lactobacillus acidophilus liquid or capsules and plain—not sweetened—yogurt. If the natural products do not restore order against the Candida army, a prescription medication can wipe out the invaders. Once this has been done, excess weight often goes with them.

Hypoglycemia (Low Blood Sugar)

Known more for undermining victims with weakness, exhaustion, faintness, and depression, hypoglycemia now turns out also to be a frustrator of weight loss regimens. Dr. Langer thought he had made an original discovery that hypoglycemia can wreck a weight loss program, when he stumbled upon a writeup, "Low Blood Sugar Can Make You Fat," in the *Encyclopedia of Common Diseases*.

The article stated that filling the bloodstream with refined carbohydrates brings on reactive hypoglycemia. Blood sugar drops precipitously, so the victim downs a candy bar or a cup of coffee to recharge herself. The article describes the hypoglycemic as an individual who is tired, miserable, and hungry all the time—a perfect candidate to gain or retain weight.

Stephen Gyland, M.D., of Jacksonville, Florida, reviewed case histories of 600 solidly documented hypoglycemics and found that their five foremost symptoms are nervousness (94 percent), irritability (89 percent), exhaustion (87 percent), faintness-dizziness-weakness (86 percent), and depression (77 percent). All of these conditions would stimulate overeating. Dr. Langer soon learned that when hypoglycemia was eliminated, invariably his patients' weight dropped by up to twenty or thirty pounds.

Hypoglycemia can be corrected by avoiding certain negatives: all forms of sugar, candies, cakes, pastries, pies, dates, raisins, macaroni, spaghetti, white rice, sweetened soft drinks, alcohol, coffee, and processed cereals, and by ingesting six small meals daily.

===================== *Food Allergies* =====================

Sometimes eliminating foods to which you are sensitive or allergic can help you lose just the amount of stubborn poundage that never before yielded to your best dieting efforts.

Dr. Langer noted losses of between fifteen and fifty pounds in eighty-four patients whose food allergies were detected and eliminated. Along with the unwanted poundage went dry, scratchy throat, generalized itching, headache, rashes, sneezing, sniffling, stuffy nose, and wheezing.

In addition to foods as culprits in allergies and consequent weight gain or retention are environmental elements such as exhaust fumes, fumes from gas stoves, cleaning solvents, gasoline, animal danders, molds, and pollens.

Anybody can perform the Coca test, which will reveal food sensitivity or allergy. Invented by Arthur Coca, M.D., the test is based on a connection he discovered between food sensitivities and allergies and an increased pulse rate. If after eating a certain food, your heartbeat accelerates by twenty or more beats, the cause is very likely a sensitivity or allergy to that food.

Dr. Langer explains how to take the Coca test, during which you test one suspicious food at a time. Find the spot on the inside of your wrist where you can feel the pulse of your pumped blood. Count your pulse for six seconds, then multiply that by ten to learn what your resting pulse is. In an extreme case Dr. Langer saw the pulse of a patient rise from 72 to 180 after she ingested an allergenic food.

Some patients have spared themselves the lengthy testing of every food they eat by eliminating the common foods to which many people are allergic. Dr. James Braly, a disciple of Dr. Theron Randolph—perhaps the most famous living clinical ecologist, offers his list of the most frequently offending foods and beverages: beef, chocolate, citrus fruit, coffee, corn, eggs, malt, milk, nuts, pork, potatoes, soybeans, spices, and tomatoes.

Eliminating food sensitivities and allergies is not a common way of reducing or controlling weight, but it works uncommonly well, says Dr. Langer.

Stress

Exhaustion of the adrenal glands—one of the key systems for coping with stress with their fight or flight mechanism—through regularly repeated, persistent, and long-enduring stressors can cause you to overeat, to gain weight, or to remain overweight. Many individuals are not even aware that they are draining their adrenals, just like they drain the battery trying to start a car with a bad ignition.

Many stressors are so subtle that it is hard to realize they are helping to deplete our adrenals. Patients are not always aware of how devastating this is to them, although they tell the doctor of their jitteriness, anxiety, depression, and overeating.

The following are twenty-one manifestations of overstress:

1. Cold hands (despite normal thyroid function or properly supplemented thyroid).
2. Eyestrain (nervous blinking).
3. Gritting or grinding the teeth.
4. Frequent headaches.
5. High blood pressure.
6. Shallow or irregular breathing.
7. Irritability.
8. Nervous jittering of leg or legs when seated.
9. Frequent finger tapping.
10. Either increase or decrease of appetite.
11. Decline of sense of humor.
12. Loss of interest in sex.
13. Insomnia or frequent waking from sleep.
14. Oversleeping.
15. Upset stomach.
16. Difficulty thinking.
17. Excessive drinking or smoking.
18. Abuse of tranquilizers.
19. Tenseness.
20. Ceaseless anxiety.
21. Feeling of insecurity and inadequacy in the face of circumstances.

According to Dr. Cary L. Cooper, professor of organizational psychology at the University of Manchester (England) Institute of Science and Technology and an international authority on occupational stress, identifying your specific stressor or stressors is important, because it can contribute to remedial action. You can often enlist help or cooperation from people who may not even realize how they are stressing you. Other corrective measures he recommends are running, sauna, and biofeedback, which get rid of the symptoms of stress until you can cope with the specific stressors.

It is important to reduce pressure on yourself by learning

how to make proper adjustments to stress, because stressors can impair digestion and assimilation, diminish benefit from food, and, as a result, cause a greater craving for food and a nonstop appetite for foods you don't really need to satisfy the body.

Control your reactions to stressors and you will control your appetite and eat reasonably, and reduce weight or maintain yourself at the desired level.

Heavy Metals

Usually, heavy metals that stealthily invade our bodies—lead, cadmium, and mercury—are considered ravagers of good health or silent assassins, but rarely, if ever, are they regarded as the cause for adding or keeping on excess weight.

Dr. Langer tells about a patient named Evelyn, a short, plump, thirty-fivish homemaker, who asked for help with her black depression, intermittent pain in the liver area, low blood sugar, and overweight.

Evelyn confessed to eating "nonstop."

Asked about her diet, she said it was about 70 percent refined carbohydrates and the rest protein and fat. Dr. Langer touched her in the liver area and she cried out in pain. The liver was definitely enlarged and inflamed.

Could the condition be fatty degeneration? Could Evelyn be a secret alcoholic? Asked how much she drank, she responded directly and sincerely, "hardly ever."

Evelyn's low-protein diet, which did not include choline or methionine and included little vitamin C, apparently was contributing to a liver disorder, which very likely accounted for her low blood sugar and ravenous appetite.

Dr. Langer feared for her because, although the liver has amazing regenerative powers, liver inflammation and swelling frequently lead to fatty degeneration, the step before cirrhosis.

Suddenly the doctor began to wonder if some environmental poison was stressing the woman's liver: a chemical, a drug, an insecticide, a weed-killer, or a cleaning solvent like carbon tetrachloride. He queried her on these possibilities.

As she began thinking, it occurred to her that where she

lived might be important. For some ten years now, she had lived in an apartment at the border of the city's commercial area. She told the doctor that her apartment house was directly behind a large service station.

It was as if lightning had struck Dr. Langer. He remembered facts of a study made in a Switzerland town some years earlier, in which cancer of many types, including lung or liver, was found to be almost epidemic in houses along a major highway that bisected the town. The incidence of cancer seemed almost negligible in residents whose homes were several hundred feet from the road. The conclusion of the study was that car exhaust, laden with lead, was the major cause.

Even though little leaded gasoline could be obtained in the United States anymore, Evelyn had breathed in enough lead to make her physically ill. A hair analysis made by a reliable laboratory confirmed the doctor' suspicion. She was carrying an alarmingly high load of lead.

Dr. Langer recommended that she move into an apartment in a nearby residential area, away from congested street traffic. He put her on a diet high in complex protein—80 grams daily—with 5000 mg of vitamin C, 50 mg of B-complex, 25,000 I.U. of vitamin A, 600 I.U. of vitamin E, and three 1200 mg-lecithin tablets for their choline and methionine. She was ordered off all junk food.

The new regimen agreed with her, for she was already feeling better at her doctor's appointment the next week. She hardly noticed the pain in her liver area and admitted to feeling far less depressed.

Five weeks after her first office visit, Evelyn found another apartment in a residential area and in the appropriate rent bracket. Her liver responded to the new diet; it was now almost normal size. Meanwhile, the vitamin C was transporting the lead out. Dr. Langer saw her again two months later. She was elated about having lost fourteen pounds, merely by getting rid of the lead in her system.

Other heavy metals—cadmium, copper, and mercury—present in inordinate amounts may not only do damage to various organs of the human body, but can also make *you* heavy.

Although copper is a necessary nutrient in minute amounts,

neither cadmium nor mercury has any business in the body. Cadmium, which can upset the body's blood sugar economy and contribute to weight gain or retention, can be withdrawn from the body by a 1000 mg intake of calcium daily. As a matter of fact, calcium helps clean lead out of the system as well.

Mercury and other heavy metals can affect the liver, disturb the blood sugar balance, and even depress the immune system. Although there are pros and cons, one group of dentists advocates getting rid of amalgam (mercury-containing) fillings and replacing them with harmless nonmetallic materials. Amalgam fillings are made of silver and anywhere from 35 to 50 percent mercury.

Mercury, like other heavy metals, harms the liver and contributes to overeating. Dr. Langer advises his patients to have their amalgam fillings replaced if possible. The cost is high, but good health is worth something too—as is being able to keep your weight down or under control.

Now that you know the ailments that may be blocking you from losing weight, you can do something about them—something constructive.

CHAPTER SEVENTEEN

HOW TO BEAT CELLULITE, THAT BUMPY FAT!

. . . So they did eat, and were filled, and became fat . . .
Nehemiah 9:25 (KJV)

*I*N I Thessalonians 5:18 we are told in no uncertain terms, "In everything give thanks . . ."

It may not be the world's easiest thing for you to give thanks for cellulite if you're in great shape with one glaring exception—you've got saddle bags that could ride the pony express. Unfortunately, they're riding your thighs instead, camouflaging an otherwise terrific figure and giving you a conspicuously lopsided look.

There's a mystery about cellulite (pronounced "SELL-u-leet," if anybody cares). I'll never know how it escaped being a four-letter word. Neither will the 80 percent of women over fourteen who have some, as estimated by James Braly, M.D.

According to Dr. Gary Friedman, head of plastic and reconstruction surgery at French hospital in San Francisco, the term "cellulite originated in France and describes the 'cottage cheese'-like appearance of certain skin. The tendency towards cellulite seems to be familial and can develop as early as the teen years. It is present predominantly in women and most commonly seen on the thighs and buttocks where fat accumulations are the greatest and is generally progressive into old age."

A controversy still rages as to whether or not cellulite is regular white fat or some other variety, despite the fact that scores of comparative microscopic studies of tissue structures and bio-chemical analyses have shown it to be white fat, arranged and distributed in a way that no respectable fat would tolerate. "Mic-roscopically," says Dr. Friedman, "fat from an area with heavy cellulite appears no different than any other." So, in theory getting rid of it should be no more of a problem than ridding yourself of the usual white fat.

That's theory for you!

There are two types of cellulite, soft and hard. Generally, women have some of each. Of what is it composed? Supposedly fat, body wastes, and water. Its origin? Supposedly toxins: air pollution, other environmental pollutants, junk foods, additives in processed foods, medicines, chlorine and fluorides in water, food allergens, incompletely digested foods, and poisons from wastes retained too long in the lower intestines.

The best-selling book of ten or fifteen years ago, *"Cellulite" Those Lumps, Bumps and Bulges You Couldn't Lose Before*, by Nicole Ronsard, lists factors contributing to cellulite: fatigue, insufficient water intake, lack of proper exercise, polluted air, shallow breath-ing, poor blood circulation, poor eating habits, sedentary living, and tension. These factors produce constipation, poor circulation, and sluggish digestion.

A medical condition that could also contribute to these three disorders is hypothyroidism (low thyroid function). With insuf-ficient thyroid hormone, the heartbeat is not strong, so blood is not pumped in force to all body cells. Likewise, constipation is a major symptom of hypothyroidism. Thus body wastes accumu-lated through constipation could become part of the cellulite com-plex.

Is cellulite common only to overweight persons? No. In my aerobic dance classes, I have seen many slender 105- and 110-pound women with this problem. Cellulite picks its victims in-discriminately.

Granted, cellulite is an almost universal problem. So why is there almost no research on how to cope with this disorder? The answer is both simple and unsatisfactory. It is not a killer con-dition, although it can embarrass a woman to death. Researchers feel there are more pressing research areas to pursue. Women do not unanimously agree.

Because experimental information on cellulite is almost non-existent, I have studied the subject for many years, starting with myself and interviewing women and preventive medicine specialists who have managed to overcome this condition.

In my earlier years, as I mentioned in the first two chapters, I began to develop cellulite in the buttocks area. Thinking that this was attributable to being overstressed, living on coffee fixes, eating junk food, and rarely exercising, I began reversing my indiscretions and living with connectedness to God.

Within less than a year, the cellulite disappeared. And the only cellulite I have seen since then has been on other people. Many women who have succeeded in ridding themselves of this unbeautiful fat and many doctors who have helped patients do the same have actually used a program somewhat similar to mine.

Let me elaborate. At that time I was dealing with basics: losing weight and rejuvenating my body. Cellulite was only a minor consideration. My reasoning was that in connectedness with God, you try to live as near as possible to the earth and conditions as He provided them for us: air, water, food, and security based on the clear knowledge from the Scriptures that he has made provision for all of life's requirements.

About that time my husband and I moved to Atherton, California (not far south of San Francisco), where our home was surrounded by a virtual forest: towering eucalyptus, pines and giant oaks, and a paradise of shrubs and flowers. It was a joy to breathe deeply the oxygen that the trees, shrubs, and flowers provided. We were also near enough to the ocean for clean salt air.

I did deep breathing exercises and was thankful for the health benefits I was getting right from God with every breath I took. Since those days more than twenty years ago, the whole field of psychoneuroimmunology has exploded with evidence that adding the mental and spiritual dimensions—by imagination—contributes powerful reinforcement and physical gains.

Then I joined a gym—this was before they became health clubs—and took classes in spirited daily aerobic exercising for an hour. Feeling the tingle of blood circulating to parts unknown, I just imagined the good that vigorous exercise was doing for me.

Sometimes I would bicycle into the hills of Atherton in the

bright morning, enjoying grey squirrels frisking around the oaks, an occasional red fox darting across the country road, and a cloud of yellow butterflies moving toward me. These exercise and nature excursions again connected me with God.

And in the water I drank and the food I ate, I sought connectedness, too. No more chlorinated tap water for me, I resolved. I had read that many vitamins (A, B, C, E) and the amino acid tryptophan were destroyed or at least reduced in effectiveness by chlorinated water, and that it also caused allergies and even brought on asthma attacks in susceptible people. Knowing that chlorine is a main ingredient in bleach, I said, "That's it. Only bottled mountain spring water will be drunk in this house from now on." So it was. Again I imagined the benefits the family and I were gaining from this move.

Then, too, to remove impurities that had accumulated in my body over the years, I stepped up my water drinking from six glasses daily to nine. Many authorities feel that such a move is necessary to detoxify the body. I don't know how much this did for my cellulite, but how much better I felt!

And I did the same thing with food, finding a farmer's market with freshly picked produce and going on a vegetarian-fruitarian diet for a few months (including a protein supplement), which ensured regularity and purged accumulated poisons.

As a result of all these changes, not only did I lose the desired weight, I noticed that the cellulite had disappeared. I don't miss it a bit. Now that connectedness is a way of life for me, I know cellulite will never play a return engagement on me.

When I feel the urge—and I often do—I eat only lightly cooked vegetables for breakfast: beets, rutabagas, and turnips. This fare seems to purify me and connect me with God. (Again, a powerful faith makes it so.) On physical, psychological, and spiritual levels I then feel even better.

After my lectures so many women ask me for my anti-cellulite regimen that I'll present my "Menu for the More Determined Dieter" just after this chapter. (Too short to be a chapter, it will be a chapterlet.)

Dr. Gary Gordon recently reinforced a deeply held conviction for me when he said, "The mind is still the greatest healer the body has." I began to utilize this healer powerfully in my war against both fat and cellulite, and found I could use my imagination to help accomplish my goals. Traveling in the realm of imagination is intrinsically healing because it demands a certain level of relaxation. Your imagination is a piece of psychological space where you can monitor the rumblings of your subconscious mind; it is also a theater in which to rehearse behavior. If you can imagine something, you can do it. When you imagine something using as many of your imaginal senses as possible, you create a real psychological event.

If you were to imagine a voracious, angry bear within arm's distance ready to spring on you, your heart would race fast and furiously, your breathing would become shallow, and your palms would begin to sweat—all signs of physical terror.

Your body is where you will be living for the rest of your life. Isn't it time you made it your home? More important, the Scriptures tell us that we are the temples of the holy spirit and that God dwells in each and every one of us—that means our bodies.

Back in the center stage realm of imagination with our bodies. Pretend you received the announcement that Jesus Christ was returning to earth and would spend his stay in your home. Begin to imagine not only the degree of diligence you would apply to cleaning drapes, windows and rugs (I need new ones), but the meticulous diligence you would apply to every nook and cranny. See yourself cleaning the floors of closets all the way to the back, cleaning long neglected drawers of every speck of lint, scrubbing dirt from under sinks.

Now, consider that the Scriptures tell us we are "the temples of the holy spirit" and that Christ dwells in us. Suddenly the unsightly accumulation of bunchy, dimpled, irregular fat on those hard to reach places—upper thighs, tummy, and hips—seems less tolerable. We can now address it with renewed zest and determination. For me this took the form of first freeing myself of fears and anxiety by living one day at a time. Matthew 6:34: "Have no anxious thought for tomorrow, for tomorrow will have thought for itself. Sufficient unto the day is the evil thereof." I stopped borrowing trouble from tomorrow, my main cause of stress. Fear and stress turn down the flow of our vital juices, interfere with digestion and assimilation, and make us live ten-

tative, cramped, fearful, defensive, fractional lives. Such negatives contribute to the dissonance of our organs and body systems
and the accumulation of toxins, which appear to underlie the
deposit of cellulite.

Mentally, I was making important choices: how I choose to
feel about my body; what kind of body I choose to have. I now
saw these as choices, not givens, and I chose to be in control.

One of the most important aspects of choosing transformation, as I was doing, was that my feelings in and about my body
were really what counted here, not the way my body looked from
the outside. Focusing on the outer form of your body makes you
an object of yourself. It takes you outside of your body. I was
determined to do spring "housecleaning" from within. I was determined to be an immaculate dwelling place. With this image in
mind there was no more place for cellulite than there was for dirty
closets.

As I drank water I began to visualize these ugly marbles of
fat being dislodged and washed out of my body. As I ate God-
made foods I could see them replacing the dead fatty cells with
lean, alive, and healthy ones. Preceding each aerobic class I closed
my eyes for two or three minutes while stretching and asked the
holy spirit to target those areas still to be cleaned and sweep them
free.

In the theater of my mind I rehearsed situations in which I
would apply various means to conquer temptation. I adhered to
the diet of Daniel, which is contained in chapter 20, "Menu for
the More Determined Dieter," and I was careful to always supplement it with free-form amino acids so as not to sacrifice lean
muscle mass and suffer protein deficiencies. In my many-dimen-
sional approach to cellulite recounted earlier, I added a filip to
the regimen.

Before aerobics I would take six 24-free aminos, two B6, and
5000 milligrams vitamin C. Remember, the body responds to two
primary commands to cleanse wastes and build cells. My theory
was that vitamin C is driven into the cells during strenuous exercise, thus aiding the body in the first of its most strategic functions. In the second strategic function amino acids, as the building
blocks of the cells, helped me to build lean muscle mass cells,
aided by a product designed for this called. I was not alone in

my internal housecleaning. My cellulite vacated the premises never to return.

Other negatives give rise to cellulite too—smoking, alcohol, junk foods, and canned and packaged foods. Smoking vandalizes the heart, the arteries, the skin, and the body's ability to throw off wastes. Consider the following:

1. Smoking contributes to cardiovascular disorders by narrowing the arteries, limiting blood supply to the struggling, oxygen-starved heart muscle and thus restricting delivery of oxygen and food to all body cells.
2. While nicotine stimulates the heartbeat, creating a greater oxygen demand, the carbon monoxide in tobacco reduces the blood's ability to carry oxygen. This is built-in suicide.
3. Constricted arteries caused by smoking minimize delivery of oxygen and nutrients to all body cells, weakening body organs and systems against attack by disease. They also make for an old-looking, lined, leathery skin.
4. Severely narrowed arteries also limit the throwing off of body wastes, a possible contribution to the deposition of cellulite.
5. Toxins from smoking are one more poison with which the body has to cope.

Alcohol depletes certain nutrients—vitamins B-1 and niacin and the mineral magnesium, among the majors—and eventually causes fatty liver, cirrhosis of the liver, and consequent liver malfunction, undermining the body's glucose use system. Furthermore, a limited-service liver is an impediment to ridding the body of toxins.

One of alcohol's most damaging acts on the body is interference with the conversion of essential fatty acids to GLA and DGLA, the precursors of prostaglandins, which are short-term regulators of many body organs. In depleting the body of many nutrients, alcohol contributes to the accumulation of pyruvic acid, which when not convertible to a fuel remains a body poison and a possible contributor to cellulite.

Like alcohol, junk foods are depleted of their enzymes and make a great demand on the pancreas to produce more enzymes than it can make without stress. Also, these devitalized foods have lost most of their B vitamins, which are required for proper metabolizing of carbohydrates. Trying to get nutrients out of junk foods is like attempting to derive heat from burning wet wood— lots of smoke and little fire. Smoke is the garbage of incomplete combustion. Likewise, toxins are the garbage of incomplete metabolizing of carbohydrates. Many authorities feel that this condition can contribute to the formation of cellulite deposits.

To a lesser degree canned and packaged foods offer the same problem without a good solution. This is why I omit them from my anticellulite diet and from the Bible diet as well. Emphasis must be put on the freshest foods possible. Relevant to this, I ran across an article symptomatic of the times from the food section of a large newspaper. It's title was "Fresh Uses for Stale Bread." No comment!

So much for my approach to the cellulite problem. There are other approaches some of which make sense, and you should know them as well. Many authorities claim that massaging the cellulite works, if it is done gently and persistently over a fairly long period—that is, months. This is a low-cost procedure if you do it yourself. It is high-cost if performed by a masseuse, masseur, or massage therapist, but it might be worth the effort because pros know how to get the best and quickest results.

Now, even massage therapists have told me that massage is not foolproof but that it does work on some women. Gloria Sung, a massage therapist of San Mateo, California, puts it this way:

"Massage is a viable form of therapy for cellulite, if combined with healthful diet and an aerobic exercise program. The diet should be rich in high water-content fruits and vegetables. It should eliminate coffee and alcohol. Of course, smoking should be eliminated."

Most massage experts suggest starting cellulite massage gently, in a circular manner. "A special type of massage is necessary," says Gloria Sung. "This is a deep, connective tissue massage— vigorous on the lumps and fatty deposits."

Also, exercise instructors have informed me that spot reducing is not foolproof in doing away with cellulite, even though cellulite is supposed to be white fat. You can't be sure if it will work or not.

Some experts say that with nutritionally balanced meals—
no specifics from them—and a brisk exercise program over many
months, cellulite disappears along with the usual deposits of fat.
It certainly did with me, but I know the superfresh foods—fruits
and vegetables and whole grains—had a lot to do with that.

Christine L. Wells, Ph.D., professor of exercise science at
Arizona State University, seems to have a good idea what cellulite
actually is. She says that it's not a different kind of fat but an
aggregation of fat cells supported by connective tissue structure,
and there's little or nothing you can do about it but perform low-
intensity exercise and follow a low-fat diet.

Wells states that women seem to have more cellulite than
men because they are generally fatter. When men gain enough
weight, they get their fair share of cellulite, too. When you lose
weight, you lose at the same rate all over.

Many authorities feel that cellulite is caused by inner pollution interfering with microcirculation, which results in the deposit of wastes, body fluids, and fats in various places. Smoking
and alcohol, much coffee, insufficient intake of water, inadequate
diet, and stress contribute to this pollution, which can only be
corrected by eliminating these negatives.

A recent poll states that 48 percent of women would opt for
a cosmetic surgical procedure called "liposuction" to remove the
bulges. Dr. Gary Friedman, head of plastic surgery at French
Hospital in San Francisco, whose results qualify him as an expert
in this art, states:

"Liposuction is neither a panacea for being overweight nor
a substitute for diet and exercise. It will never make a fat woman
thin. It's a refining process during which one or two pounds of
excess padding is removed from a specific area of the body to give
an otherwise fit body better balance and contour. The healthy
woman with inherited excess fat may find it practically impossible
to achieve her ideal body image with diet and exercise."

"Let me offer a few qualifiers," says the handsome, dapper
surgeon. "If you're overweight, can't stick to a diet or exercise
program, or see surgery as an end-all cure to your problems,
liposuction is not for you. It's major surgery and in the hands of
an unqualified surgeon, mix in a poor candidate, and horrendous
and dangerous, even deadly complications can occur.

"Once fat cells are removed they never grow back. However, chronic overeating will cause remaining fat cells to expand. In any case, eating properly is essential to maintaining the results of liposuction. The best candidate is someone who is of normal weight, is in good physical shape, follows a good diet, and exercises regularly to maintain muscle and skin tone. This person has inherited deposits of fat that no amount of diet or exercise will get rid of. Good skin tone is essential because once fat is removed, the skin must shrink down to fit a new contour. Skin that lacks elasticity will form unsightly ripples, waves, and irregular contours. But good skin tone is more a result of a moderate life style than age. Factors like excessive sunlight, smoking, and drastic shifts in weight can decrease skin elasticity, while regular exercise, proper diet, and slow weight loss can enhance or restore skin tone. I routinely find that older women who exercise regularly have better skin tone than younger women who don't."

Cellulite seems like a problem that can't be solved. Yet it is being solved beautifully every day by the methods described in this chapter.

CHAPTER EIGHTEEN

LOVE THYSELF AND LOSE WEIGHT

For as he thinketh in his heart, so is he . . ." Proverbs
23:7 (KJV)

*T*HREE beautiful, shapely young women, 20 to 36 years of
age, could never have been expected to love their neighbor,
because they didn't love themselves, particularly not after the
severe setbacks they suffered.

Blond Robyn, 40, a former runner-up in a beauty contest in
one of the southern states, came to Hollywood on the promise of
a top talent agency to start her small and build her big. She started
small. That was all.

Pert, vivacious Ellen-Rae, 30, had flown out to San Francisco
from Des Moines, Iowa, to marry that Dream Man, a key executive
with one of the Fortune 500 companies. Strange. No one was
waiting to meet her at San Francisco International Airport. When
paged, she checked at the airline desk and found a "Dear John"
note from her Nightmare Man.

Auburn-haired, 36-year-old Jan, with that smart, tailored look,
had been a model before meeting her husband-to-be. She "modeled" him through medical school, internship, and his start in
private practice. A society doctor, he practiced his bedside manner
in many a mansion and eventually ended up in one of them with
a multi-multimillionairess.

Now the postscripts.

Blond Robyn, disillusioned, depressed, too embarrassed to

return home a loser, hung in there in Hollywood, worked as a waitress, and wrote glowing letters about her prospects in films and TV.

Ellen-Rae couldn't go back to Des Moines without a husband. So she picked up a series of odd jobs just to keep going until she found herself another dream man.

Jan couldn't very well leave the scene of her humiliation and go home to mother. Both she and her mother had lived in San Francisco for ages.

From here on the three different stories merge like tributaries into the main stream. Their self-esteem badly battered, the three women began flogging themselves with self-defacing questions: "Where did I go wrong?" "What do you do when life is all over?" "What's the use?"

Little by little the pattern of negativity and self-pity began to take over, and they ate a little more than usual to soothe the pain. And as the years went by, those extra ounces of food added up to many, many pounds. And, now, each one hundred or more pounds overweight, they had a new problem to add to their rejection: a burden of fat, a waddling walk (especially embarrassing for a former model) and an inability to walk any distance without being out of breath. And the crowning humiliation: obesity, which limited them socially and in their careers and reduced their chances of marriage.

Does that sound like curtain time of Act Three?

Don't you believe it!

These women sought secular and Christian counseling, and realized the solution to their problem wasn't in eating their way into a new set of problems but in starting from the ground up: reconstructing their stressed and strained self-esteem.

Every one of them is now a success, having lost the unwanted poundage and having succeeded.

Robyn owns and operates one of Southern California's smartest restaurants, patronized by many of the stars.

Ellen Rae sharpened up the feminine charms that had won her the attention of the executive in the first place. She began attending a Christian church, where she met and married a widowed owner of several thriving entrepreneurial firms.

A new, slender Jan visited a friend in the hospital. There,

outside of the room, she ran into the president of the hospital, a man she had known and admired for years. He had admired her for years, too. They are now engaged to be married.

These three women did things the hard way. They could have reprocessed their self-esteem right after their personal disasters and avoided the defeatist overeating.

The first thing they could have done is the most difficult of all: after the tears, they could have become objective about something subjective and concluded that what happened could have happened to anyone. The second thing they could have done is admit that they had had a crushing blow but that they could weather it as they had other serious crises before. The third thing is not to have felt sorry for themselves. An investment in self-pity is one of the worst you can make. It leads to something worse—if that's possible—self-condemnation and loss of your prize possession: the healthy self-esteem that is a necessity for survival, good health, and happiness.

Another typical negative development is turning against the person who maligned you and letting hatred, resentment, and the desire for revenge corrode your insides. So one person or set of circumstances has given you a sharp setback! This does not prove that you lack self-worth. Believe in yourself as you did before. Others do.

You are going to start out all over again and come out better than ever. So if you need a new outfit to repackage the new you, all right. Treat yourself. It's a positive step.

I know what I always do when it seems the world has sat down hard on me. I remember who I am. God made me, and He is noted for doing an excellent job. I am a child of God. With God and His vast power, I am an army. I won't let God down by feeling sorry for myself—not for an instant. I will use the physical, mental, and emotional resources God gave me and, despite a setback, work with His help to improve them. If what I lost seems precious, I know that with faith in God I will find something even better suited to me and my needs.

These words remind me of what happened to an acquaintance of mine I'll call Kent. Kent had been attending National Health Federation meetings in the San Francisco area for as long as I was president of this organization, and we had had many chats between sessions.

He had been hired many years before as the manager of a breakfast and lunch restaurant by a more or less absentee owner, a man who operated numerous enterprises. At one time the owner had promised that in five or ten years, he would give Kent half interest in the restaurant for his loyal service and creative ideas, which have made it one of the most thriving restaurants of its kind in the area.

One of Kent's innovations was offering health food alternatives for clients as well as the usual fare. Another was offering to pack special, cold but appetizing lunches for office workers as they ate breakfast. These lunches were packed flat to fit into attaché cases, so that executives wouldn't lose face by carrying a brown bag.

A year had gone by since I had last seen Kent, and as I spoke from the platform, I noticed in the sixth row, right in line with me, a man who looked familiar yet unfamiliar—a person so beefy that he strained the buttons of his vest and seemed uncomfortable. I almost gasped when I realized it was Kent.

"What has happened to him?" I asked myself, still holding to the pattern of my talk to the audience. Then I answered myself, "What happened to him was a good sixty more pounds."

It was difficult to wait until the intermission. Finally, we found a quiet corner where we talked and drank herb tea together. Shortly after our last San Francisco convention, Kent had learned that the restaurant owner was retiring. He had reneged on his promise to give Kent half ownership and had installed his 25-year-old son to co-manage the place.

"With this frustration and the son getting in the way, all I seem to do is eat," Kent confessed. "I can't sue the owner, because it's against Christian principles."

"Can't you get a cash consideration instead?"

"Yes, $35,000, which is just a fraction of what half ownership would be."

"Why torture yourself?" I asked. "Take it and run. You don't want to work with the son anyhow."

"No."

"Remember that great idea of a new type of food service you mentioned last year? Why don't you start it with the capital you'll have?"

Hope gleamed in Kent's eyes again. "I've been feeling too sorry for myself to think constructively."

I learned Kent had been demoralized when, on top of his business problems, his wife had called him a "loser." Obviously, he had little self-esteem left. I prayed a silent prayer for an idea that might help.

All that came was to tell Kent to get back to his basics—to realizing that God is his source of supply and that we should depend upon Him to furnish opportunities through people. I asked Kent to study just one flower in his garden—the intricacy of design, the manifold details, the distribution of color—to remind himself how God takes care of his works of art like the flower and his other works of art like us, if we rest in faith with Him.

Kent came back the next day all recharged.

So did I. I told him about one of my friends who owns a large food supplement firm who had just lost his executive vice-president and corporate expansion genius through death. I suggested Kent tell my friend his idea for his novel food service. (It is impossible for me to reveal the nature of the business without violating a confidence.)

We three had lunch a few days later, and the president of the food supplement company loved Kent's idea and wanted to put it into practice at once. Appreciation made Kent's self-esteem expand, and he poured out a torrent of related ideas. The meeting brought about one of those made-in-heaven matings of men and ideas.

Kent is now executive vice-president in charge of corporate expansion, making twice his previous salary with commitments for stock options and freedom to develop his numerous plans. Happier than he has ever been, Kent and his wife have reconciled. He has already lost forty of the sixty superfluous pounds and is his wife's "thinner winner."

Do you remember the title of this chapter? "Love Thyself and Lose Weight." That is the key. If you begin to lose self-love, you soon begin to gain weight. Not a very good exchange.

The Bible Scripture at the chapter head reads: "For as he thinketh in his heart, so is he . . ." To win at weight loss, you've got to think thin. You can if you love yourself—and you must love yourself because that is basic to being able to love God and your neighbor.

Let me accentuate the negative for just a minute. Fat people think differently about food than thin people do. They even think about food when not hungry. They anticipate three meals a day even when full after the first meal. Food is almost always a part of their social life.

Food is more than a mere way to nourish the body in time of hunger for fat people. Any time is hunger time. Eating is an emotional experience, a way to soothe unhappy feelings—hurts, slights, frustrations—and to celebrate happy ones.

A towering reason why most weight losers can't retain their new slenderness is that they keep their mental image of fatness. Therefore, the old eating habits must return to conform. Only a famine can restrict such a person.

Conversely, a person who thinks thin won't be inclined to be fat under any circumstances. So the mental image of thinness must precede diet and exercise.

Changing from a fat to a slim state of mind can be agonizing because it involves breaking the iron grip of the eating process as the primary source of comfort, solace, and gratification, and facing up to problems, troubles, and needs. This is a revolutionary change for anyone who has spent a lifetime avoiding such a confrontation.

The very stress that such a changeover causes can trigger the desire for high-fat foods, as indicated by a scientific study described by my biochemist friend, Luke Bucci.

Gopi Tejwani, a researcher at Ohio State University, showed that when white mice were subjected to high-level stress, they developed an overpowering hunger for foods high in fat. Tejwani found that stress caused the brain to release chemicals called beta-endorphins. When he injected the white mice with a substance that blocked the beta-endorphins, they lost their cravings for fat foods.

A similar biochemical action takes place in human beings,

but we presumably have a greater mental capacity to deal with stressful situations than the white mice do.

If the seriously overweight person is shy and is among strangers or people he thinks don't like him, he feels the pressure of the situation. The "fat" thinker overcomes this stress by eating. He doesn't have to carry on a conversation if his mouth is full.

On the other hand, the "thin" thinker usually doesn't fear other people. She will initiate conversations, ask others about themselves, listen to what they have to say, and follow up on each hint or lead the other person offers, pursuing the new acquaintance with the curiosity of a child. The natural fear of what is unknown is replaced by the feeling of warm comfort that comes with the familiar.

A famous psychiatrist made a confession to me as we shared adjoining seats on an airplane flight. "I used to take copious notes about my patients. Then one day I discovered that they always reveal themselves and their troubling problems within the first half hour. Everything that follows is redundant."

The thin thinker, also, has found that people are easy to get to know.

The fat thinker has her own way to cope with the pain of daily living. It often differs from that of the rest of us. Many of us feel that a certain amount of pain and trouble come with the territory, so we acknowledge and then shrug it off. All of us have felt betrayal or suffered some hurt at the hands of others.

However, the fat thinker has learned that there is no pain, trouble, problem, feeling of insecurity, or dirty trick for which food and the process of eating food cannot be a soothing comfort. Yet she actually sees through the comfort as only temporary, because after the sunny gratification comes the terrible aftermath of gloom, the intense feeling of self-contempt, because nothing has been solved.

The thin thinker has learned to deal with problems directly rather than take a food anesthetic, perhaps praying like St. Augustine for the ability to change those things that can be changed, for the strength to endure those things that cannot be changed, and for the wisdom to know the difference.

Ultimately, thinking thin is a matter of getting down to the bone of who and what you are: your self-esteem. Down deep you must find a lovable and worthy person. To lose weight permanently, even if it's just several pounds, you must love and accept yourself—even your fat—for exactly who you are.

You must be able to accept your basic lovableness without sham or reservation. The problem of being overweight may stem not as much from what you are eating as from what's eating you. Do you dare face your pain, your vulnerability? Or do you seal yourself off from your feelings? If I have learned anything in life, it is that life requires a price if you want to be as fully alive as you can be.

You need courage to pursue the truth of your life and yourself. Is it wrong to love yourself? Of course not. Jesus commands us to do so when he tells us "to love one another as we love ourselves." If we can't face up to and learn to accept and love ourselves, how then can we possibly accept others? And how can we expect them to love and accept us?

How can we integrate ourselves so we can handle life's problems as they come at us? How can we find out our strongest motivation? Sure, we all know about survival, but we go beyond that and end up with self-acceptance and self-love.

Knowing that God created me and has authored some quality things is my starting point. Then I take it from there. I have certain characteristics: love for God, integrity, honesty, friendliness, a caring and love for others, a sense of responsibility, a degree of creativity, ability to conform to laws of God and man, and the moral courage, when the facts justify, to take an opposing stand on important issues.

If you are short on self-esteem, you may have gnawing at your subconscious mind the frightening fact that you were born with more fire, more vitality, more creativity, more perceptiveness, and even additional special gifts, but you haven't expressed them as much as you should have. Some children are especially endowed with such gifts.

Rare gifts such as these can make a youngster seem a rebel, an oddball, or a nonconformist to other kids, parents, and teachers, particularly in a social environment where pressure is applied to stampede us all to conform.

At this point the youngster must make a choice: to be a rebel and use his talent—to be ahead of his time, and to become a leader rather than a follower, or to give in to the fear that such a choice will make him or her unacceptable or unlovable.

A great deal of fat can suppress such potential. Then you hate yourself—damage your self-image and self-esteem—because in the inner recesses of your soul you know that you are being untrue to yourself.

Or maybe you are on the other side of the fence. Perhaps you are one who has tried desperately to please others—first your parents and then your spouse, children, boss, co-workers, friends, relatives, or neighbors—without regard to what pleases you.

By the time your suppressed desires express themselves in eating for psychic gratification and you become fat, you may not even realize or dare to recognize that you are smouldering within for having spent so much of your life trying to please everyone but yourself. At a deep level of consciousness you know that you are not the person you want to be.

Of course, there's nothing wrong with pleasing other people, but it is hardly the prime directive of life. The Scriptures advise us to "live our lives as under the Lord, and not as under man." The thin thinker does not live his or her life to please other people, but does, nevertheless, bring pleasure, satisfaction, and brightness into the lives of others.

Food is so tightly knit into socializing that what I am about to say may appear to be too nonconformist, but here goes anyway. The acid test of lovableness to ourselves and to others will come when a friend visits and, instead of food, you give her the gift of joy in her own being. Feed your friend with the milk of human kindness by giving your complete attention and acceptance—an honor and a novelty in today's society, where people think of their next remark instead of listening to what others are saying.

So many times fulfillment comes just from having someone who will listen and reach out a hand to say, "I'm sorry." This can be the turning point from emptiness to rich experience. Remember that man cannot live by bread alone. And the nurturing you can give will be remembered and appreciated far beyond the fattening calories you have to offer, no matter how deliciously prepared.

The results will be twofold: while enriching your friends'

lives with your sincere interest and questioning, you will gain the deep reassurance of knowing that just you are enough.

What could be more uplifting for your sense of self-esteem than to know that you fulfilled without offering other than the finest gift you have—yourself? As you multiply this, you will find that you become a welcome guest and a trusted friend, because you showed interest in what people think of as the world's most fascinating subject—themselves.

How do you show your interest in others? Learn to question them and really listen and hear. Follow every lead that's given. Ask about their work: Do they like it? How has it affected their personal lives? What is their hobby? Could it ever become an avocation? A full-time business?

Such interest is essential for total aliveness. Through allowing others to be all that they are capable of being, you become all that you can be: real, sensitive, caring, honest, willing to give and express feelings of vulnerability.

Once you have achieved these things, you will find that you have that love of self, that self-esteem, that gives you the strength and courage to overcome whatever sense of guilt, fear, rejection, or frustration has led you—ounce by ounce—to being overweight.

You will feel that strength come through in a strong determination to fulfill yourself and your potential rather than fill your stomach and suppress your individuality. When we think fat, we restrict ourselves socially and in employment, and we dig a grave for ourselves with our mouths. One pity-filled thought leads to another until the only difference between a rut and a grave is the depth. But now we have stopped this vicious cycle. Now we are thinking thin. Now we are beginning to celebrate life.

With renewed respect for ourselves, we can become aware of our bodies and the foods we put into them. We eat to live, not live to eat. And inasmuch as we eat to live, we should become more concerned that what we do eat gives us nutrients needed by our bodies for good health and excludes those things that do us harm.

We have too much respect for ourselves to consume either the quantity or the quality of food that destroys our quality of life and, with it, ourselves!

CHAPTER NINETEEN

USE FAITH TO LOSE WEIGHT

If ye have faith as a grain of mustard seed, ye shall say unto this mountain, remove hence to yonder place, and it shall remove, and nothing shall be impossible unto you. Matthew 17:20 (KJV)

*F*AITH can move mountains, including mountains of fat. I didn't have actual mountains to lose, but they certainly weren't valleys.

Some years ago, I asked God for an instantaneous weight loss miracle, but He didn't give me a miracle. He gave me something better: the basis for faith that eventually led me to my Golden Secret for weight loss and weight control—not only for myself but for you.

As mentioned in chapter 1, my Lake Tahoe experience thrilled me and supercharged me with faith. Twilight time quietly arrived—a time of lengthening shadows—and I was awed by the splendor of the God-given setting: towering, majestic, green pines lining the lake shore; the clear, glasslike water; and the clean, bracing air and silver stars beginning to glitter.

The thought struck me then that God had hung the stars in space, that He had formed the earth and spun it into orbit, that He had created the magnificent scenery all around me, and that He had also created the person in the center of that scenery—someone, as Psalm 8:5 states, "a little lower than the angels."

I thrilled at God's omnipotence, omniscience, and omnipresence until chilling goose bumps rose on my arms. To such an all-powerful God my weight was no problem. All I had to do was put everything into His hands and sustain my faith in Him. And with such faith would come the Golden Secret in stages: KEEPING CONNECTEDNESS TO GOD AND HIS NATURAL FOOD SUP-PLY, AND BEING COMMITTED TO A MENTALLY AND PHYS-ICALLY ACTIVE LIFE SERVING GOD AND MAN.

That was exactly what I did. Consequently, I am now slender. For the past ten years there has been almost no fluctuation in my weight. I no longer even have to think about it. My life of faith has dissolved that problem.

Here's how the secret came to me. First, God told me to get rid of unnatural foods, that is, man-made, and eat only foods as close to the way He made them as possible: whole grain cereals, fish, some eggs, dairy products, small amounts of meat, all the garden-fresh vegetables I wanted, and moderate amounts of fresh fruit—never anything canned.

I followed His instruction to the letter. And what an uplift of the spirit when you live by the Master's Plan! It seems more revelations follow when you not only believe but also have the faith to take the first steps in the right direction.

It occurred to me that I probably wouldn't have been rein-troduced to natural foods—my mother had first introduced me to them—if it hadn't been for my friend Helen's illness and my efforts to help heal her. A verse from Romans 8:28 became real to me: "All things are not good but all things work together for good to them that love God to them that are the chosen according to His purpose."

Another key development sprang from Helen, too—a cause so all-consuming that I hardly had time to think about eating, let alone eating. I was driving Helen to Albany to see John Richard-son, M.D., in hopes that laetrile, a natural therapy he adminis-tered, might still save her. It was too late, but while in Dr. Richardson's waiting room I talked to many patients who had been given up for dead by the medical orthodoxy and who, with Dr. Richardson's laetrile treatments, were now stopping by just for a checkup on the way to the golf course.

Helen's death and that of others showed me how bankrupt traditional medical treatment was for cancer: surgery, radiation, and chemotherapy, which patients in the waiting room referred to as "cut, burn, and poison."

During that period nothing was being done to prevent cancer. It was traditional medicine's stance that doctors are trained to treat symptoms not to prevent causes. While a river of gold was being poured yearly into cancer research, deaths through the scourge of cancer only continued to mount, and it seemed all the funds were being appropriated to refine the techniques of "cut, burn, and poison." While buildings and personnel were added each year to cancer research organizations and budgets and overhead expenses mounted astronomically, cancer deaths continued to rise to 485,000 annually.

This tremendously costly counter-punching troubled me. One of the ironies was that the American Cancer Society was formed in 1913 as a temporary organization to be dissolved when cancer was cured. All I read in the press was how worthless laetrile was, and all I saw in Dr. Richardson's waiting room were people who were being healed with this "worthless" form of therapy. Orthodox medicine had the press in its hip pocket and was using it to damn laetrile, and while deaths continued to escalate the FDA and AMA absorbed themselves, their energies, and their resources (your resources really) to block simple, God-given, low-cost therapies. Could that be because the FDA costs for getting a new drug approved run a minimum of $90 million? I began to see the FDA as a protection racket for the drug industries, persecuting and prosecuting simple, natural, gentle therapies because they couldn't be patented. No one is going to invest money to have a substance approved when they cannot receive a return on their investment.

Then one day, with full television coverage, Dr. John Richardson's offices were invaded by the state food and drug representatives. This benign man was manacled to his nurses and hustled with them out of his suite like a criminal. This police-state act was perpetrated with patients left on gurneys, IV needles still in them, with no one to care for them.

The crime Dr. Richardson had committed was daring to use an alternative form of treatment. It mattered not that laetrile was harmless and had, after all, cured some people. His sin was in not conforming to the bankrupt "cut, burn, and poison" philosophy which was producing rapidly increasing death statistics each year.

Incensed about Dr. Richardson's humiliating treatment, I started a newsletter among his patients to raise money for his legal defense and to fight for the right to use alternative forms of cancer treatment.

For many years previous to that I had been immersed in the simple wisdom of the constitution, its veneration of the individual and its constraints on the machinations of government. I revered its astonishingly straightforward and sensible construct of law and limited government, which used not many more words than I will in this chapter. I observed that it did not confer upon Americans any rights whatsoever, as it acknowledges that man's rights come from God and not government. It is a document of "enumerated powers" that quite specifically defines the duties of government, chief among which is to secure for men those rights they already possess. I was greatly influenced by the constitution and its authors, who recognized fully the untrustworthy nature of men in positions of power and so established rule by law, not by men. As Thomas Jefferson said, "In questions of power, then, let no more be said of confidence, in man, but bind him down from mischief by the chains of the constitution."

For years I had been trying to motivate my fellow Americans to understand that we are a society under attack, whose collective liberty is endangered because everyone's individual liberties are threatened. The war against freedom has been going on since the dawn of civilization, I would pontificate yet, because America is the greatest example of freedom embodied in nationhood. America is the undisputed battleground upon which a life and death struggle plays out every day before eyes that are educated to see it.

From my understanding of the constitution, it was obvious to me and as meandering of government through the swamp of socialist thinking over the past seventy or eighty years attests, as events both recent and historic at home and abroad make abundantly clear, the responsibility for the defense of this nation, its people, and its liberty belongs to those who understand both the blueprint and the building.

In championing the cause of freedom of choice in medical care, I was taking a most important single step toward the defense of our liberty. And defend it we must, against Communism from within and without and against Big and Bigger government. The American people trusted the medical establishment; they felt the FDA was protecting them against quackery. To that I offered them number 25 of the Federalist Papers, written by Alexander Hamilton: "For it is a truth which the experience of the ages has attested, that the people are always most in danger when the means of injuring their rights are in possession of those of whom they entertain the least suspicion."

In my newsletter I stated clearly and often my conviction that as long as a person is not free to put into his own mouth what he needs to save his own life he is not free. He is a slave.

An informed cadre of supporters, one dedicated to the study and appreciation of these principles, was necessary to the support of my newsletter, and support it they did. At $10 per copy, we managed to raise $8000 for Dr. Richardson's defense. I worked free of charge, and what a blessing to know that while my labors were saving lives in many cases, they were also securing the blessing of liberty to ourselves and our posterity.

Eventually, Dr. Richardson was freed. The next move by the state was to bar the shipment of laetrile into California from Mexico. The fact that some people were being healed by laetrile did not matter. It was not an accepted, recognized treatment. That was what mattered. This struck a deep cord within me from my studies of the Scriptures. I know that God taught not only by what the Bible said but by what He did, and in the first book of the Scriptures He gave us free choice, the right to be wrong if we so choose.

I walked in faith. Using my newsletter to present the modus operandi for each individual state to carry through legislation, I lobbied in each of the fifty states for freedom of medical choice legislation. We managed to score in twenty-seven states—some of them passed legitimate bills; others adopted Mickey Mouse, watered-down, better-than-nothing measures. The remainder of the states preferred the monopolistic course even though many of the legislators had lost relatives and friends through cancer treated by traditional methods. After all, 80 percent of the congressional and state legislators receive AMA donations.

It seems God's hand was in the newsletter, because the management at San Francisco radio station KEST read it and invited me to host The "Totally Yours show." Through the various scientists and doctors I was able to bring on the air, many revolutionary breakthroughs in preventing illness and healing disease, nutrition, and weight loss and control were given a hearing. Without alternative opinion you have no free choice. I felt I was doing my part in ensuring that choice.

Meanwhile, the National Health Federation of Monrovia, California, an organization formed to fight for freedom of choice in medicine, had seen my Richardson newsletter and invited me to start a publication that would expand to a national scale what I had been doing locally for Dr. Richardson's cause—no, for everybody's cause: yours and mine. I called it *Public Scrutiny*, and it eventually merged into the NHF's present monthly magazine, *Health Freedom News*.

Somebody must have liked the work this female David was doing on Goliath, because I was invited to run for the organization's presidency. I prayed for God's guidance, but not receiving a clear response, decided not to campaign for office. I wanted to make sure He was in this with me. My answer came with unanimous election by the board of directors and then by the membership. I have served in this capacity for nine years at this writing and continue serving.

The National Health Federation applies a three-pronged strategy in laboring to keep your freedom to choose. We:

1. Educate
2. Legislate
3. Litigate

Every day those who would take away your freedom to choose are on the move, and every day they are met with determined resistance by *your* National Health Federation. Many of the freedoms we now enjoy were won for us by this valiant group of patriots.

One of our many major legislative battles was a fourteen-year struggle to keep the American Medical Association, the Food and Drug Administration, and the multibillion dollar pharmaceutical industry—the Unholy Trinity—from making vitamins and minerals prescription items.

The whole premise of this proposed legislation was ludicrous. Physicians study a minimal amount on the subject, and their official position was that vitamins are unnecessary—"all anybody needs for good health is a well-balanced diet." Yet they were supposed to be the ones to decide whether you and I need vitamins and prescribe them at their discretion.

Fortunately, legislators saw in this power move an abridgement of freedom of access to an important adjunct to health, which is almost as important as freedom of the press.

As I write, after building a bulwark of support on the federal level, the dieticians are attempting an end run by moving to pass legislation in each state to force all nutritionists to take the necessary courses to become credentialed. On the surface this seems a legitimate move; the only problem is, these so-called professionals study the traditional medical school idea of nutrition, whose crowning achievement is debilitated hospital food. They should only be sentenced to eat the so-called meals they create for hapless patients.

Again, this is a power grab that would force the nation to accept the brand of nutrition that brings on deficiency diseases and that would limit advice health food store workers can give customers without the workers ending up in prison. This one comes close to ending freedom of speech for health store owners and workers unless they were degreed with the orthodox credentials. Technically, you wouldn't be able to advise your family or neighbors on matters of nutrition.

Your freedom of choice to have fluoridation in your water enforced at the federal level would have been violated were it not for the National Health Federation. Also, were it not for the NHF stopping an Orwellian thought-police bill sponsored by the late Senator Claude Pepper in 1980 and again in 1984, you would not be able to obtain material through the mails or by any other instrument—that means radio, TV, newspapers, or your own car—that goes "against the weight of scientific and medical opinion." Remember, the Bible goes against the weight of scientific and medical opinion.

It would also be illegal for a dissenting book such as this to be written. There would be no room for dissent. Only credentialed party-liners would be able to write for publication, and should these writers veer from the party line, they could lose their credentials. This "thought police" technique would limit alternative information, indirectly censor information that the public should receive, and reduce the quality of health—good business for the drug companies but not for our good health. It would be like suppressing a Semmelweis*, a Lister or a Pasteur. (That's progress!) Innovation in information would be dead and embalmed, along with health enhancement through prevention.

The incredible part of this is that several states, not seeing the picture in proper focus, have bought this package and have passed legislation for credentialing nutritionists.

During one of my never-ending battles for health freedom came a turning point in my career. My daughter Colleen, an expert in phone selling, was confined to bed at home, recovering from an auto accident. She secured me a guest appearance on TV 42, Family Christian Broadcasting, in Concord, near San Francisco. I had made sporadic TV appearances before. I was to be on the network's flagship program, "California Tonight," hosted by Ronn and Connie Haus, the owners of the station, who have since become my precious friends.

I talked about my book *Nutrition: the Cancer Answer* on the show, and audience response was so enthusiastic that the producers, John and Kathy Fitzpatrick, came up with the idea of my hosting a health interview show. I was asked to call John and Kathy within a few days to confirm availability. Wanting to get God's approval of what I was doing, I never phoned back. Finally, John phoned and said, "Hey, Maureen, you were supposed to call back."

They had seen me as a guest on one of the highest rated Trinity Broadcast Network shows, "Calling Dr. Whitaker" an Angel Award winning health interview program hosted by Donald Whitaker, M.D.

Then Paul and Jan Crouch—Paul is president of Trinity Broadcasting Network (TBN), the largest Christian network—in-

---

* *Semmelweis was a nineteenth-century Hungarian physician who reduced mortality from infarction in childbirth by insisting that doctors and attendants on obstetrical cases wash their hands thoroughly. He was ridiculed for this procedure, which was accepted as standard practice 36 years later.*

vited me to be a panelist with Dr. Whitaker and Dr. Robert Mendelsohn, best-selling author, on a nutrition program. Enthusiastic listener response motivated TBN to feature my 30-minute "Accent on Health" show twice weekly on TBN's national and international network.

Looking back, I see that both my weight and my career problems were solved through prayer for guidance, learning to relax and trust in God's provision, and moving ahead on faith.

Faith really works, as illustrated by the following stories about Jack Hanley, Rose Ann, Lynda, and a woman whose name I do not know.

In the San Joaquin Valley, Jack J. Hanley, with the support of his devoted wife Lillian, was legendary for hard work, honesty, and integrity. Impressed by his parents, their young son Jack L. was eager to emulate them and their deeds. Measure up, he did, adding working smarter to his parents teachings. His upwardly mobile career escalated with the force of a hurricane—so much so that by the age of 28 he kept 15 phones busy racking up $8,000 in phone calls a month, and he was making more money than the chairman of the board of Dean Witter, the brokerage firm for which he worked as a commodities broker and where sheer grueling hard work had won him the title "King of Cotton." He had won his own laurels, carved his own image, become his own legend. His successes were perhaps even more far reaching than his father's, and they were in the sophisticated world of high finance, a world of high highs and deep depths.

If you had the misfortune to be trading against him (as often happens in commodity trading) he was a formidable power to be dealt with. If he was investing for you, you could comfortably unload your burdens on his broad and capable shoulders.

Jack Lee Hanley is possessed of a golden aura. At 6'1" he is tall, handsome, and courtly. Long sweeping lashes frame vivid, piercing blue eyes. His long romanesque nose makes his luminescent face almost angelic. He is no dilettante. He captured the hard-won respect of his coworkers by being willing to do anything he had to do to get the job done.

"I got up with the chickens and went to bed with the owls," he says. By the time the other workers arrived at the office at 7 A.M. Jack had been there since between 3 and 5 A.M. and was halfway through his day. Sometimes he wouldn't leave at all. Sleep was the only luxury he could not afford.

Jack's passion for work had a down side, however. The consuming demands on his time seemed to leave him with no time for nourishing meals. It was difficult enough to get out of bed before dawn, much less plan that extra hour of morning time that breakfast stole from an already overtaxed schedule. Cigarettes, stored conveniently in his desk drawer, could be smoked without distracting him from a proposal whose details engrossed him into the late night hours. Perhaps later on he would find time, he might promise himself. For now, coffee to awaken, cigarettes in the office, and a drink in the evening to make him feel lively would have to do.

Coffee with sugar, sometimes as many as twenty cups, from 5 to 11 A.M. had to sustain him. By the time he left the office he had smoked two packs of cigarettes. He left the office anywhere from 2 to 9 P.M. to entertain clients, many times eating steak, potato, and lettuce salad at nine at night.

A decline by degrees into heavy alcohol dependency seemed to happen without notice. Many times he would go directly from the bar to work. While he remained faithful to his workload, he seemed to be functioning on automatic. As 1970 progressed, alcohol no longer sustained him along the starkly unreal schedule he had set for himself. Unable to snap back from the nightly binges, he tried pot, at first to accommodate a friend and then to accommodate himself. Marijuana, it seems, didn't leave the hangover that alcohol left. What it did do was cause a voracious appetite. The munchies plagued him. While the pot seemed to mellow him out, the craving for snacks that followed was incessant. A fast-food restaurant across the street provided him with artificial milk shakes that settled brontosaurus-like on his belly. His weight climbed from 170 pounds to 215 pounds.

In an attempt to conquer the munchies, he found that cocaine was a useful tool in suppressing his appetite. He then began to take all three: alcohol, marijuana, and cocaine.

From that point on, the depression that surrounded him created a malaise of relentlessly darkening days and relentlessly lengthening nights. He had to find a way out of the cul-de-sac of his life.

Under the stress of his frantic, nerve-jangling profession, he continued to overeat and underexercise. Somehow he felt that if he could stop all his addictions, he could lose about thirty-five or forty pounds, particularly in the belly area. But his nerves were ragged from the frantic daily pace of trading, so he couldn't stop drinking, putting away half a quart of vodka daily, and he continued to both smoke pot and take cocaine.

"It seemed hopeless to try to do away with my habituations," says Jack, "let alone lose weight too. I had to find a way out of the web I had found impossible to extricate myself from alone. Then a friend patiently began to explain to me that even while I was a hopeless sinner, God had sent his son to die for me. She opened the Bible and showed me example after example of how God loved me on the basis of His character not mine.

"It was not difficult to convince me. It was the answer that satisfied the longing in my soul. I felt connected beyond our solid sphere. It gave me the fulfillment I needed to be able to do away with my habituations, to face all my troubling addictions, including my weight."

Nothing consequential seemed to happen immediately, but then, as the days flowed by he felt either no desire for alcohol or a mild aversion to it. And he lost the longing for cocaine, although he kept being drawn back to cigarettes.

"I didn't sweat it," Jack admits. "Then one day I smelled the old, dried-out contents of an ash tray and nearly gagged. That was it!"

Along with losing his desire for alcohol, cocaine, and cigarettes, Jack Hanley began to lose fat—almost forty pounds in seven weeks.

Faith has also worked wonders for others. Rose Anne (not her real name) had a wonderful pinkish, smooth-skinned cherub face, but she carried at least eighteen pounds more than she needed. Every diet published seemed to help her lose six or seven pounds, but that was it.

Once when she was down seven pounds, an attractive businessman named Phil began to show interest in her. No matter what she tried, she could not get the last ten pounds to budge. All she had to show for a new strenuous daily exercise program was sore muscles. Rose Anne became sick at heart with frustration. One evening her businessman arrived early, detected tear-stained eyes, and questioned her about them. She confessed the reason.

"You look great to me," he responded, "But if you want to lose, let's pray." So they knelt and prayed together that God would accomplish what Rose Anne couldn't.

When Phil stood up, he told her, "Rose Anne, within three days from now, weigh yourself. You will see a marked decline."

Eagerly Rose Anne waited for the third day. Finally, it arrived. As she stepped on her bathroom scale, the indicator traveled ahead, then stopped. She had lost three pounds!

"It's a mini-miracle," Phil exclaimed.

And it was. Those last seven pounds rolled off like the first three. Even though Rose Anne had tried everything she could not get cooperation from her body, but she believed enough in a miracle that one came to her. Phil had spoken the word of faith, and what Rose Ann felt was that a miracle had taken place.

Lynda had a peculiar problem. Only a matter of five pounds separated her from ecstatic happiness. But where the pounds were located was her source of embarrassment: in her belly.

"I looked pregnant all the time," she says. "Most women collect fat on their hips or thighs, where they can hide some of it. But me? I could have died with embarrassment."

Exercises worked to a degree, but she still had about three pounds to lose. "Why not go for a miracle?" her girl friend Renee asked.

"How?" Lynda asked. "I don't know any miracle workers."

"Jesus," replied her friend.

"No," she responded. "He's dead."

Renee replied, "Oh, no. Hebrews 13:8 says, "Jesus Christ, the same yesterday, today and forever."

Renee and Lynda attended an Assemblies of God church in the San Francisco Bay area. As Lynda knelt at the front of the church, the preacher, in vestments, laid hands on the top of her head.

"It felt as if cracked ice were moving down from my neck through my body," Lynda confesses. "I could literally feel my stomach go down, as if it had deflated. Now I'm as flat as a board. What a miracle!"

Recently I met a woman who had slimmed down to 140 pounds from 435 pounds. "I'll never be fat again," she told me with such certainty that I believed her.

Burning with curiosity, I asked, "How did you manage that?"

"Through the Scriptures. I didn't realize that through incessant eating I had made food an idol. Without realizing it, I was practicing idolatry, placing food above God. This devastated me, so I determined to put God where He belonged—first."

The woman told me that this Scripture powered her through the crisis: "Know ye not that ye are the temple of God and that the Spirit of God dwelleth in you? If any man defile the temple of God, him shall God destroy; for the temple of God is holy, which temple ye are." (I Corinthians 3:16 (KJV)

She reminded me that most obese individuals develop physical ailments from their overweight. "I was so motivated, I prayed to God for forgiveness for my idolatry and asked His help in placing Him first and honoring the body temple He had given me."

"How long did it take?" I asked.

"I started two years ago and it is still going on. Now I eat only for nourishment. God has helped me put food in its proper place. I lose a pound or two a week."

When I lecture to women's groups, particularly, I tell them that if their faith is smaller than a grain of mustard seed, they can develop greater faith by reading and memorizing certain Scriptures.

Hebrews 11 is the great faith chapter. Whenever I need faith for a miracle, I reread some of these Scriptures. The following good parts always ignite and excite me about possibilities:

From Hebrews 11:6–9 (KJV):

"But without faith it is impossible to please him: for he that cometh to God must believe that He is and that He is a rewarder of them that diligently seek him.

"By faith Noah, being warned of God of things not seen as yet, moved with fear, prepared an ark to the saving of his house: by which he condemned the world, and became heir of the righteousness which is by faith.

"By faith Abraham, when he was called to go out into a place which he should after receive for an inheritance, obeyed; and he went out, not knowing wither he went.

"By faith he sojourned in the land of promise, as in a strange country, dwelling in tabernacles with Isaac and Jacob, the heir with him of the same promise."

The best is yet to come—the parts about the city with foundations and Abraham's wife Sarah having a baby at an extremely advanced age:

"For he looked for a city which hath foundations whose builder and maker is God. (Hebrews 11:10)

"Through faith also Sarah herself received strength to conceive seed, and was delivered of a child when she was past age, because she judged him faithful who had promised." (Hebrews 11:11)

I recall, after a lecture in Denver once, giving the above Scriptures to one of the heavyset women who surged around the speaker's stand. I thought no more about it, and several years later I was lecturing in Denver again. There was something familiar about one of the women who wanted a minute of personal chatting.

"Remember me?" she asked with a slightly self-conscious laugh.

"You do look familiar."

"You just don't recognize me because when I was here several years ago, I weighed eighty pounds more."

I was awed at the trim youthfulness of this lovely woman. "How did you do it?"

"Don't you remember? You gave me a sheet of Scriptures from Hebrews 11. I memorized them as you recommended. Once they were almost indelible in my brain, I began to have real faith. These things were not just lines in Scripture. They had actually happened. My faith rose high."

Fascinated, I asked "Did you ask to lose certain specific poundage?"

"No, just to lose the spirit of gluttony. All I used to do was eat, think about eating, eat more, and think more about eating more."

"Thank God."

"Exactly," she replied. "I lost my lust for food. I soon had a moderate appetite. The weight came off at about two pounds a week."

One of my favorite miracle-working Scriptures is Matthew 17:20, which I'll quote in part:

". . . If ye have faith as a grain of mustard seed, ye shall say to yonder mountain, remove ye hence to yonder place, and it shall remove, and nothing shall be impossible to you."

I keep this scripture pasted on the bathroom mirror, on the refrigerator door, and even on the desk where I work. The impossible is always possible when I reread this scripture.

Keep remembering that this is God's promise and that He keeps His promises.

Expect a miracle, but don't try to make God conform to the exact specifications of the miracle you want. He may offer you a Scripture that will help you. If it is a Scripture, write it out on a piece of paper and memorize it and believe in it until it becomes a part of you.

Speak the words aloud. I have seen some nearly miraculous weight losses by people who spoke the Word. The excess weight seemed to ease off during a night's sleep and the appetite just seemed to shut down.

The age of miracles is still here!

Take advantage of it!

DANIEL'S MENU FOR THE MORE DETERMINED DIETER

J RARELY lecture anywhere that people don't ask me how I stay slender. The answer is a simple one. I advise it, however, only for the more determined.

When I do find those highly motivated and disciplined few, I can guarantee them weight loss of two pounds a day.

I eat no sugar or refined flour and drink no caffeine or alcohol. For breakfast I lightly steam a pot of root vegetables. My favorites are beets (with the leaves) and turnips. I sprinkle on an herbal seasoning and eat as much as I want. This is so filling I feel little impulse to snack. If I do feel inclined, I will have an apple or other fruit.

For lunch I have a vegetable salad to which I add water-packed tuna or an egg. Vegetables in the salad predominate, and if I use lettuce I make certain it is of a more rugged variety so that pesticides have been kept to a minimum.

Throughout the day I drink bottled water with lemon. From noon to 1:00 P.M. I take an advanced aerobic class. This regime has consistently allowed me to lose one to two pounds a day. I stay on it until I lose the desired amount (usually that last six pounds).

As part of this regimen I take a supplement program of 24

free-form amino acids, fortified by the addition of tryptophan and carnitine.

Amino acids have been said to be the royal flush of protein digestion. They deliver the end-product of protein digestion to the cells. I like to call them organized protein.

These amino acids, particularly trylophan work in still another way, reducing the sensation of hunger, as explained in a recent workshop by Dr. Lindsey Berkson. Tryptophan is used by the brain to produce serotonin, a neurotransmitter that sends out messages from the brain, such as "You've eaten enough."

This is why "Bears don't eat honey 'til they pop. They seem to be satiated at a certain point," explains Dr. Berkson.

The lovely bonus I have enjoyed from these products is that as a result of taking them to preserve lean muscle mass and therefore more effectively burn calories, I have doubled the density of my hair. My hair stylist first noticed the small sproutings when they were an inch or two in length. I was so pleased by the new luxurious thickness that I have grown it shoulder length for the first time since I was a teenager.

Here is my total supplement regimen:

4 multivitamins (two after breakfast, two after lunch)
2 50-mg B6 tablets taken each morning with amino acids to help their transport. B6 also reduces edema (excessive fluid in tissues).
24 free-form amino acids, including carnitine.
2 tablets of a natural plant growth factor that helps the body increase lean body mass.
4 digestive enzymes with meals. These contain betaine hydrochloride and natural bromelain.
5 drops of vitamin A-E emulsion. A and E should be taken together so that both can be properly assimilated. This emulsion has returned a glowing moisture to my skin.
4 to 6 500-mg evening primrose oil tablets (2 to 3 after breakfast and two to three after dinner).
6 to 8 1000-mg vitamin C capsules, 3 to 4 after breakfast, 3 to 4 after lunch. An important antioxidant, vitamin C plays a critical role in muscle and bone integrity, strengthening the adrenal and immune system func-

tions, and serves as a protective agent against infection
and degeneration.

3 500-mg bioflavonoids (rutin) to contribute to capillary integrity. Biochemist Oscar Rasmussen, Ph.D., recently
stated on my TV program that bioflavonoids also have
an estrogen-like activity.

Minerals To ensure the proper amount of minerals, I take a
solution derived from clay deposits of vegetation origin
containing 70 major and trace minerals in proper balance. I take one ounce twice daily.

Individual nutrients in such a program are balanced and
harmonized like the various instruments in a symphony orches-
tra. They thus tend to keep the metabolism in balance, burning
calories efficiently and keeping excessive body fat from accumu-
lating.

CHAPTER TWENTY-ONE

THE MOST ASKED QUESTIONS ABOUT WEIGHT LOSS

. . . And when the wise is instructed, he receiveth knowledge. Proverbs 21:11. (KJV)

A SUPER low-calorie bit of wisdom comes from Proverbs 18:20 in the Living Bible: "Ability to give good advice satisfies like a good meal."

Oh, to be that caliber of advice giver! Refrigerator doors would open far less frequently, dresses would not fit so tightly, and bathroom scales would be much more complimentary.

I'm not always sure that my weight loss advice to those who respond to my TV program satisfies me like a good meal, but the questions are superb, representative of what most people are eager to know.

Let me give you the most often asked questions and my answers to them which are based on dozens of reliable sources. (They cover all phases of weight management from diet to behavior modification to exercise.)

1. *QUESTION:* It seems all I get is invitations to birthdays, parties, showers, weddings, bar mitzvahs, and anniversary celebrations, and there's food, food, food everywhere—food that undermines my best intentions and my latest diet. How can I cope with this curse?

ANSWER: Well spoken. We all have to deal with this one. What works best for me is eating at least a partial meal before I attend a party, the kind of meal in which I select the foods, so that I can keep the calories as low as I please. Then, at the party I do token eating. (Nobody ever told me not to eat the tokens.) Most party fare is loaded with calories, so I just go through the motions. Even at that, I eat mainly vegetable sticks and avoid the tasty but calorie-laden dips. Don't let yourself be vulnerable! Rule one is, never come hungry, because then it's hard to resist the wicked stuff. Rule two is, always hold a munchie in your hand, so that you don't get strong-armed by somebody insisting that you "Try some of this!"

2. QUESTION: My Achilles' heel is restaurants. I do well at home, where I can control my caloric intake, but, Maureen, at restaurants all my good deeds are undone with too-big portions, salads swimming in dressing, crisp, perfectly browned rolls baked on the premises, and that vulgar but wonderful display of French pastries? What should I do?

ANSWER: My heart goes out to you, but not my sympathy. I love to try new restaurants, but that doesn't mean I relinquish control of my calorie counts when I dine out. No way! I pay the bill, so I call the shots. First, I use my local restaurant guide or articles from weekend sections of newspapers to steer me to places where they serve various-size portions, so I can order exactly the amount of meat I want. Then I have the salad dressing served on the side so I can use as much or as little as I wish. About those crisp and perfectly browned rolls, I will have one with fresh cream-ery butter—just one! Inasmuch as I try to limit eating out to once a week—it doesn't always work—I permit myself a bit of recre-ational eating. But at that French pastry, I draw the line. One portion has tons of calories and many nutritional "No-nos," so I resist the Napoleons. I'm no cream puff!

3. QUESTION: In times of emotional stress, I'm afraid I let myself eat when I shouldn't and consequently pack away too many calories. I can ruin my diet for a week in a single meal. Usually one of the foods, such as ice cream, can drive me into binge eating that you wouldn't believe. How can I turn myself off when emotional states turn me on?

ANSWER: Join the club. Those of us who are not easygoing are subject to eating pressure when we're depressed, joyous, excited, lonely, frustrated, or overtired. Knowing how susceptible you are to your emotional states gives you an advantage. Take an iron grip on it. You also appear to know at least one of the foods that trigger you into a binge: ice cream. Instead of letting your negative and positive emotions push you into eating—taking in extra calories—let them push you into exercising—burning up calories. Also, the exercising, if vigorous enough, will dissipate the power of these emotions. Then *you*, rather than your emotions, will be in control. Make a list of all your binge-promoting foods and avoid them.

Remember, you are in charge of your vulnerabilities. They are not in charge of you.

4. QUESTION: Not long ago I read an item in our local paper headlined, "Sugar Isn't as Bad As Most People Think." Is this for real or do I detect the fine hand of the Sugar Association spreading its sweet, innocent-white, crystalline propaganda? Also, the article states that there's not that much sugar in high-calorie desserts—that it's mostly fats. Is refined sugar really so bad for me?

ANSWER: Your original assessment of the article was correct. You do detect the fine hand of the Washington, D.C.-based Sugar Association spreading its sweet, innocent-white, crystalline propaganda. Nicely stated! I have a copy of a version of the same article before me, and paragraph 3 is probably the funniest: "And, yet, for reasons not altogether clear, sugar has acquired a shady and mostly undeserved reputation in recent years."

Oh, sugar, how could they so malign someone as sweet as you? Let's face it, biochemists are beasts to reveal that refined sugar helps boost blood cholesterol levels, that a high intake of sugar, if not quickly burned, turns into saturated fat, and that sugar revs up production of alkaline digestive juices in the stomach, making calcium insoluble and contributing to osteoporosis. A high intake of refined sugar also increases the need for the vitamin choline and may in turn cause kidney and liver damage. So if there are many calories of fat in gooey cakes and pies, there is also a great deal of sugar.

One of the statements of the article is that "sugar stands pretty well acquitted." Pardon the legalism, but nobody is "pretty well acquitted." A person is acquitted or not. Based on the charges two paragraphs above, sugar should "pretty well" be sentenced to life, bowl and all.

5. QUESTION: Is it true that certain foods can make you hungry right after eating and therefore should be minimized or eliminated from the diet? If so, what are they? Conversely, are there foods that quickly quench hunger?

ANSWER: You're right on both accounts. Something I'm going to say here could just as easily have been tucked into the answer to the above question. According to research done at Yale University by Dr. Judith Rodin, professor of psychology, foods with high glucose (sugar) values—beets, bread (both white and wheat), carrots, cornflakes, honey, Mars bars, parsnips, potatoes, rice, and shredded wheat—stimulate insulin synthesis and therefore increase appetite. White bread, cornflakes, and Mars bars are not exactly the foods of which dream diets are made!

Dr. Rodin discovered that the following foods reduce appetite: dried beans, fish sticks, ice cream (make sure, ice cream isn't a binge starter for you or an allergen) lima beans, milk, peanuts, dried peas, sausage, tomato soup, and yogurt.

6. QUESTION: I vaguely remember reading somewhere that if you go on a very low calorie diet and lose weight quickly, you risk developing gallstones. Right?

ANSWER: Yes. Sixty-eight heavy patients at Cedars-Sinai Medical Center in Los Angeles were put on a 500-calorie-a-day diet. In four months they averaged a 40-to-50 pound decrease in weight. However, one-fifth to one-quarter of them who melted off fat quickly were found to have developed gallstones.

Along with the departure of excess poundage comes the arrival of greater amounts of cholesterol. This substance hardens to form painful pellets of gallstones, which must be dissolved by drugs or removed by means of surgery.

7. QUESTION: Are there ways of tricking your body into

thinking that your hunger is satiated—that you've had enough food and don't need any more?

ANSWER: Yes. You have probably tried one or two of them without thinking much about them. They are covered in some depth in chapter 22, "Banish Fat With Natural Health Products," particularly guar gum and glucomannan. Pectin also gives that "oh-so-full" feeling.

Dried beans, oat bran, and, of course, oatmeal are excellent sources of fiber. Fruits high in fiber are apples, apricots, berries, cherries, oranges and grapefruit, peaches, plums, and pears. Among vegetables, carrots and tomatoes are rich in pectin. At least eight glasses of water daily have proved helpful in making the stomach feel full, too.

8. *QUESTION:* It is my understanding that overweight people put away food much faster than the rest of us. If this is so, how can we reduce the speed at which we eat?

ANSWER: Easily, without having to put a governor on your mouth. Some individuals make a practice of deliberately alerting themselves to the slowdown by chewing the first three mouthfuls twenty times each. Once they're conscious of this, it's not difficult to reduce the speed of the rest of the meal. A second method is setting a timer for at least twenty minutes. This method actually reveals you have a motor-mouth if you finish a meal in ten or twelve minutes. Once you extend yourself beyond twenty minutes, the message has time to be transmitted to the brain that you are full. Some individuals practice gaining mastery over their appetites by putting down fork or spoon for a few minutes at a time. This, too, helps eat up the clock and produces the feeling of satiation.

9. *QUESTION:* How early in life does the habit of overeating take place? And what specific occurrences bring it about?

ANSWER: Overeating apparently starts a day or two following birth, say some authorities. Whether you were breast-fed or bottle-fed seems to be the deciding factor in a lifetime of eating normally or of overeating. Researchers in England weighed 250 normal, full-term, six-week-old babies. Sixty percent of the bottle-fed babies were overweight, compared with 19 percent of the breast-fed babies.

Certain authorities claim that the warmth, nearness, and love of the mother are so satisfying that the infant knows intuitively when to quit feeding. They theorize that the bottle is unsatisfactory and that the bottle-fed infant is anxious and stays with it longer, taking in more milk than the breast-fed infant does.

These feeding patterns persist into childhood and adulthood, with the breast-fed baby having a superior feedback system, cutting off earlier than the overeating bottle-baby, whose cut-off system is faulty. This negative pattern is worsened in childhood when parents insist that children eat everything on their plates.

10. QUESTION: Are polyunsaturated fats, like corn, safflower, and soy oil, losing favor as nutrients to control blood cholesterol levels?

ANSWER: Yes. This is touched upon in chapter 6, "Cholesterol, Weight Loss and You," showing the actual hazards of polyunsaturated oils in contributing to aging in general and to aging of skin in particular. Additionally, although polyunsaturates may reduce the bad kind of cholesterol, they often reduce the good kind as well.

Olive oil, so commonly used in biblical times, has been found by Dr. Scott M. Grundy, director of the Center for Human Nutrition of the University of Texas at Dallas, to lower harmful LDL cholesterol and raise helpful HDL cholesterol.

11. QUESTION: Is meal skipping ever a practice that pays dividends to the dieter? I ask this question because I read results of a survey showing a rise of 63 percent in the past ten years in the number of individuals who skip lunch.

ANSWER: That was a survey conducted by MRCA Information Services. Skipping lunch is a negative practice, although not quite as harmful as skipping breakfast. It often leads to low blood sugar and inefficient functioning in the face of overfatigue. In this competitive world you need all the nutritional help you can get. Elsewhere in this book, I have stated that the only meal that can be justifiably skipped is dinner, inasmuch as most individuals watch TV at night and don't need a big meal to energize them for that. It is best to have your greatest intake of food nearest the time of your greatest output of energy, as numerous experiments have shown. Skipping breakfast or lunch brings on the reactive effect. You feel abused for having been done out of what you feel is your caloric entitlement and usually make up for the missed meal with excessive calories during the next meal.

12. QUESTION: Is it a good idea to base your standard of weight on actresses and models? Or are such standards way off the norm?

ANSWER: They are usually unrealistic. Weight control authority Dr. C. Wayne Callaway, director of the Center for Clinical Nutrition at George Washington University, states that twenty-five years ago, models were some 8 percent below the average weight. Now, they are 23 percent below average weight.

Several surveys, one carried in *Psychology Today*, reveal that no matter how slender women are, they think they are fatter than they should be. So don't use actresses and models as standards. They are poor standards even for themselves. Some look bony and angular, like cadavers in the making.

13. QUESTION: I seem to be habituated to overeating and I'm not too successful at breaking out of this pattern. Just because there's a leftover piece of meat on the platter or in the refrigerator, I feel compelled to eat it. What's the answer?

ANSWER: One is to plan portions for no leftovers. You are in an excellent position. It is much easier to refrain from eating a second chicken breast when you're already full—far easier than resisting the first one. Develop your resistance. You can shatter the overeating habit in several ways: by eating the favored food until you can't stand it or are exhausted by it; by substituting another pleasurable habit—nonfood, that is—in place of it; or by tying the bad habit into a negative experience, aversion therapy (learn how to steel yourself to its unpleasant aspects).

14. *QUESTION:* No matter how I try to eat less, I end up thinking I am a victim of circumstances: at the mercy of my appetite, as if its some kind of monster detached from me.

ANSWER: I used to have that awful feeling. I won when I stopped thinking of myself as a victim of a conspiracy and visualized myself in command. When you're in charge you have more self-esteem. You're more powerful. Your appetite must take orders from you. As an overeater, you are an obsessive-compulsive person who eats addictively. Because you are a servant to your obsession, you lack respect for yourself and soon adopt a "What's the use?" attitude. There's an emotional gap in your life. You fill it with food. Find out precisely what you lack and try to fill that lack with exactly what you need emotionally—not with food, which is just a substitute for your real need.

15. *QUESTION:* Does it really matter exactly when you exercise in relation to eating? Should it be before or after or in between?

ANSWER: If it's in relation to controlling appetite and losing weight, the best time for exercising is before eating. I do it about thirty minutes to an hour before. There are some advantages to following such a program. One of them has to do with blood sugar level. Excess fuel from eating is stored as glycogen in the liver and muscles. This can be converted to glucose on demand. Exercise places a big demand on us, so the blood sugar is elevated for needed fuel. With thirty minutes of aerobic exercise, you will see your blood sugar level rise, causing your appetite to decrease. What a help in making you adhere more closely to your appropriate eating program!

Of course, the second benefit—mentioned in chapter 12, "NonExercising: The Sin of Omission"—is getting your metabolism speeded up so that it will work to burn calories for many hours afterwards.

16. *QUESTION:* Do you believe in behavior modification insofar as losing weight is concerned?

ANSWER: Yes, I do. I have seen the most positive results in so many people's lives that I'm a great believer in behavior modification. In one experiment members of a former diet program were compared for results with people who reduced on the basis of a behavior modification plan. After six months the behavior modification group lost 55 percent more poundage than the usual dieters. While the behavior modification group lost on an average twenty-three and a half pounds, the dieters lost only thirteen pounds, a significantly smaller amount.

17. QUESTION: I have heard about eating in front of a mirror to reveal the gluttony level and multiple chins—negatives to motivate positive action. What's your opinion of this sort of behavior modification?

ANSWER: It's extremely effective. As a matter of fact, I had a health authority on my TV program and later sent him a copy of the videotape. He was appalled by what he called "the gross appearance of my chins" and took immediate remedial action: slashing his caloric intake and doing daily aerobic exercising. Would you believe that within seven weeks, he looked ten years younger and was reduced to a single chin? Do you know what he does to maintain his new self? He plays that videotape every time he's tempted to overeat. Does it work? You know it! He's so grateful to me.

Now, about eating before a mirror. That works wonders, too. Several friends of mine who tried it were appalled by how they actually shoveled food into their mouths and by their washed out and often bumpy skin and—worst of all—double and triple chins. One woman told me, "Maureen, I was shocked, then almost nauseated by my appearance. I promised myself I wouldn't quit working on my inordinate appetite and deteriorated appearance until I was a new person." Now she is. The mirror behavior modification really works.

18. QUESTION: I understand that many people try substitution—a form of behavior modification—and find it successful. What I mean is, instead of gratifying themselves emotionally with food, they substitute nonfood rewards.

ANSWER: Yes, it works well, too. Try some of the following "insteads": attending a legitimate theater performance, curling up with an exciting new book, seeing a TV special, watching a sports event, bowling or playing tennis, or even doing aerobic dancing with friends. (So far as the latter is concerned, classes are held day and night.)

It may seem amazing, but forty obese persons were questioned in depth by a researcher, who found that eating was not one of their favored activities. Ahead of eating was socializing, working, and nonfood enjoyments. So substitutions will not be that hard to find. It's just a matter of making out a list of favorite enjoyments in order of preference and then following them when the urge to overeat asserts itself.

19. QUESTION: Even in exercise these days, people are trying to get gain without strain. I just heard about a researcher who administered pills to test subjects that stimulated the heart the way exercise does, to see if the patients could derive benefits similar to exercise without the sweat and strain. Is this possible?

ANSWER: The actual purpose of this was to determine whether or not people with heart disease could attain cardiovascular fitness without exercising. An experiment was conducted with dogs. Exercised dogs that were given the pill showed marked benefits. Caged dogs did not. The researcher concluded that you can't attain cardiovascular fitness by means of this drug. It has to be attained through honest exercise.

20. QUESTION: It seems that most diet books really tell only half of the story, or less, when they don't stress the need for exercise along with reduction of caloric intake. Right?

ANSWER: Right. Dieting and exercising do opposite things. Dieting slows down metabolism so less fat is burned; exercising speeds it up to burn away more calories. So it is best to combine dieting and exercise. If you have to choose just one, however, exercising is your better bet. The person who is anchored to a chair all day and thinks dieting alone is going to help him can forget it. Trying one diet after the other is doomed to failure. Each new diet is just basic training for the body to survive on even less energy—turning the metabolism way down—to require less food, and to utilize even less oxygen.

21. *QUESTION:* I understand that stress can create false hunger and motivate you to eat food you don't need. Doesn't it make good sense to dig deep and find the source of your emotional stress so that you can deal with it directly, rather than do peripheral things like exercise?

ANSWER: If your stress is clear-cut and obvious, you can then deal with it frontally. However, there are many stressors—some obvious, many subtle. Often they are overlapping and form a complex, and then they are hard enough to untangle let alone deal with. The subtle stressors can best be handled through vigorous exercise and by these other means:

1. Ridding yourself of hidden hostility
2. Crying
3. Laughing
4. Hiking
5. Confiding in a trusted friend or family member
6. Listening to music
7. Praying
8. Shopping
9. Sleeping
10. Taking a weekend off or vacationing

22. *QUESTION:* Isn't it all right to take pills that curb your appetite—if just for a little while to get in the habit of dieting?

ANSWER: Appetite suppressants (anorexians) kill your hunger and give you a big energy charge. They can even *kill* you. Physicians are only supposed to prescribe them for four to six weeks. Used in large doses over a protracted period, they can create psychic and even physical dependency, cause difficulty in swallowing, delusions of persecution, and even depression. Many doctors prefer to utilize fiber rather than pills that can be hazardous to health.

At least fiber is a natural product, with a minimal chance of hurting you. With so many different types on the market, it will be easy for you to find the one that's right for you.

23. QUESTION: Most of us girls at the country club—like so many other Californians—want to lose some poundage, so we're cutting down on fat. When I go to the supermarket I always buy low-fat milk, because I still get my calcium. Isn't that one of the best ways to cut fat intake?

ANSWER: Actually, there are many ways to reduce your fat intake, as outlined in chapter 14. Drinking low-fat milk isn't the best. You do get calcium and a few vitamins, but as recommended in chapter 14, you can do better by drinking whole milk and reducing fat in other foods.

What bothers me most about your statement is that you live in California, where you have access to the world's best milk, Stueve Raw Certified milk from Alta-Dena. The cream in this milk is rich in the Wulzen factor, an anti-stiffness nutrient discovered by Dr. Rosalind Wulzen of Oregon State University. (Controlling stiffness is something individuals should consider more as they advance in years.) The Wulzen factor is absent in skim milk and negligible in pasteurized whole milk.

Don't forget that 4 to 5 percent of natural milk's calcium is lost in the pasteurization process, along with much of its phosphorus and its vitamins C, B-2, and B-12, and 90 percent of the enzymes that help the body utilize proteins, fats, sugars, starches, phosphorus, and calcium.

Raw certified milk standards are far more rigid for cleanliness and wholesomeness than those for ordinary milk. I am pleased to say products from Stueve's are now being distributed outside of California and will soon be sold in all fifty states.

CHAPTER TWENTY-TWO

BANISH FAT WITH NATURAL HEALTH PRODUCTS

Feed me with the food that is needful for me . . . Proverbs 30:8 (RSV)

*M*AN'S subtractions from God-given foods make later additions necessary if we are to prevent declining nutrient
values, preserve our health, and keep our weight under control.

This adds up to uncommonly good common sense. So my
concern in this chapter is making up for man's subtractions by
means of dietary additions that help in losing or maintaining
weight.

One of many missing or deficient ingredients in today's foods
is fiber. It was called bulk or roughage by grandma and has a
laxative effect. She could tell whether or not you were getting
enough roughage by your process of elimination. A fiber con-
spicuous by its absence in processed foods is bran.

Fiber is one of the best dietary aids for weight loss or weight
control, because it moves food quickly through the digestive system, slows down the absorption of carbohydrates, and delays the
feeling of hunger.

Perhaps fiber is most welcome in your dietary plan because
it gives you the feeling of being full. Even before that, fibrous
vegetables and fruits demand chewing, which in turn increases
the amount of saliva and reduces food intake.

When fiber is mentioned most individuals think in terms of
bran—wheat, rye, oat, or rice. But the range of fibers breaks out

beyond the grains spectrum into beans, lentils, vegetables, and fruit.

Wheat bran rates highest in fiber content per one-third cup compared with other grains and foods in other categories: wheat bran, 6.4 grams; oat bran, 4.2 grams; brown rice and wheat germ, 2 grams. Among beans and peas the following are fiber-richest per one-third cup: kidney beans, 5 grams; navy beans, 4.3 grams; split peas, 4.3 grams; white beans, 4.2 grams; lima beans, 4 grams; blackberries, 4 grams per half cup; dried prunes (three large size) 3.7 grams; and apples, approximately 2.1 grams with skin. Of course, vegetables such as celery and carrots rate high, too.

Over and above its benefits in efficient waste elimination and weight loss, a high-fiber diet reduces the rate of colon and rectal cancers by moving carcinogens quickly through the intestinal tract. According to Seymour Handler, M.D., of the North Memorial Medical Center in Minneapolis, the high-saturated-fat and low-fiber Western diet accounts for serious colon diseases. As an insurance policy against cancer, we need to reduce saturated fat and increase fiber, he believes.

Numerous studies have found that the average daily diet contains only 15 grams of fiber, roughly half of the amount recommended by the National Cancer Institute—25 to 30 grams.

While some individuals hail fiber as a real blessing, others consider it as a mixed blessing. The latter are nearer the truth. Although fiber does reduce the number of calories absorbed, it also lessens the nutrient intake in the process. Several of my favorite biochemists have warned me about diets that advocate all the whole grains, legumes, fruits, and vegetables you can eat. This is too lopsided. It's okay to get your fiber, but don't forget other key nutrients: the protein, calcium, and iron found in dairy products and meat.

Use bran with discretion and wisdom, they say. An over-abundance of fiber without enough fluid intake can bring on dehydration and with it disorders of the digestive tract. Beware of heaping fiber indiscriminately on other foods. Add it gradually —four to seven tablespoons daily—and make sure you drink eight to ten glasses of water and/or other fluids.

Part of the advised wisdom accents the fact that an over-abundance of wheat and oat bran can bring on a nutritional deficiency. Bran has a high content of phytic acid, which combines with various essential minerals such as calcium, copper, iron, magnesium, and zinc and transports them out of the body.

However, most of the news about fiber is positive. Constipation has long been known for raising blood cholesterol levels. Free, regular, and rapid transit of waste matter through the lower intestine helps keep cholesterol levels in balance.

By what means does fiber accomplish this? An article in the *Postgraduate Medicine Journal* states that the usual cereal fiber, as opposed to bran, keeps secondary bile salt from recycling from the colon and overproducing cholesterol. Long-time ingestion of this kind of fiber is as essential as a low-fat diet in enhancing the ability to lose weight.

As indicated in chapter 13, "Don't Let Stress Sabotage Your Diet," any kind of stress may encourage you to eat more than you need. Fiber to help control cholesterol levels may reduce your anxiety about your heart and arteries and therefore contribute indirectly to weight loss or at least weight control.

The excellent British medical journal *Lancet* reported not long ago on a ten-year experiment with fiber as a preventive for heart attacks. Eight hundred seventy-one middle-aged men in Zutphen, the Netherlands, were divided into two groups: those who ate 27 grams or less of fiber each day (about an ounce), and those who ate 37 grams or more. The death rate of the men in the first group was four times higher than that for the men in the group that ate the higher amount of fiber.

Let's take a closer look at fiber to see how it contributes to weight loss. First, it contains very few calories. Second, it offers a great deal of bowel bulk. Like a sponge, it sops up a lot of water—about eight or nine times its dry weight. You feel so full, you have less temptation to overeat.

High-fiber foods are far less digestible than other foods, as an experiment by the USDA and the University of Maryland proved. Just short of 5 percent of the calories of high-fiber foods passed through instead of staying in the body. This finding was based on tests of twelve men who subsisted on a low-fiber diet for twenty-six days and then were switched to a high-fiber diet—all fresh fruits and vegetables with no grains.

All sorts of new weight loss products are filling shelves of nutrition centers worldwide. You may need information on them, because often the literature accompanying them is sketchy. Some of them provide bulk; others appear to rev up cell metabolism; and still others operate in such a way that no one is quite certain how they achieve their effect.

One of the most exciting new products is guar gum, available at almost all health food stores. Guar gum was extensively tested in comparisons with other fiber for its ability to promote weight loss. As reported in the *British Journal of Nutrition*, it received the highest marks of all.

Guar gum lessened hunger significantly better than commercially available bran, as tested over a ten-week period. Then it raised the metabolism of carbohydrates and fats—a super-plus value for the overweight and the obese. Guar gum also lowered blood sugar following meals by a good 10 percent, while blood insulin levels stayed just about the same. The researchers interpreted this as a favorable sign: that cell responsiveness to insulin remained unchanged.

During the entire ten-week experiment patients remained on their usual diet. However, they lost significant amounts of weight—a result that amazed the researchers. A bonus value was the fact that blood cholesterol levels went down markedly through the use of guar gum.

Weight loss with glucomannan, another available fiber, is not quite as spectacular as that with guar gum—it lacks guar gum's versatility—but is still excellent. Considered a new product, glucomannan is actually an oldster—older than Methuselah. And that's not just a bewhiskered cliche! Methuselah racked up 969 years; glucomannan's parent, the konjac plant of Japan, has been used medicinally for more than 1000 years.

Glucomannan's claim to fame is in decreasing appetite so that dieters can adhere to a low-calorie diet. Many preventive medicine specialists tell me it works rather well but that it has to be used with good sense. You take glucomannan, a granular product, in a glass of water. It swells to eight or nine times its dry volume and makes you feel so full that you can resist overeating more effectively.

Has this product been tested for validity? Yes. An article in the *International Journal of Obesity* reported on an eight-week, double-blind study, showing that glucomannan makes a decided contribution to weight loss. All twenty obese test subjects were told to follow their usual diet and not to change their exercise patterns. With an 8-ounce glass of water before each daily meal, they were all given two 500-milligram capsules of glucomannan or a placebo simulating glucomannan's appearance.

Individuals who took the glucomannan burned off 5.5 pounds during the experiment's duration. The placebo takers reported no weight change. Further, the glucomannan test subjects found their levels of total cholesterol and low-density lipoprotein (LDL) reduced by 21.7 and 15, respectively. No side effects were observed in those who took glucomannan.

In the interests of fair reporting, it must be stated that glucomannan escorts out some of the body's necessary nutrients as well as calories. A protective measure followed by many preventive medicine specialists is to reduce glucomannan intake to two rather than three meals daily, omitting it prior to the meal packing the most nourishment. Patients melt off weight a little more slowly, but they retain more of the needed nutrients.

Two other latter-day food supplements, L-carnitine and Evening primrose oil, contribute to weight loss, but in an entirely different way from glucomannan. Carnitine, derived mainly from the muscle meats (beef, lamb, sheep and chicken), accelerates the burning of fat. An elevated level of carnitine in the body makes body fat burn faster; a low level does just the opposite.

The human body can synthesize carnitine from the amino acid lysine, with a little help from its friends, methionine (another amino acid) and vitamin C. Men are more richly endowed with carnitine than women, which theoretically should make them able to burn fat faster.

Perhaps the male body's highest concentration of carnitine is in the testes. Research has established that the lysine-deficient become infertile for lack of carnitine.

A pertinent question pops into the consciousness: If the body can synthesize carnitine, why should we have to take a carnitine supplement?

In some individuals the capacity for converting lysine into carnitine may be limited. In others the need for carnitine is too great for them to manufacture enough. Therefore, it may be necessary to take carnitine supplements of anywhere from 300 to 800 milligrams daily. It has been found, too, that increasing intake of proteins rich in lysine and methionine, supplemented by vitamin C, can kick carnitine synthesis into high gear. In two studies, one by the Mayo Clinic, it was discovered that we synthesize some four times as much carnitine as we take in by diet.

Several experiments have demonstrated that exercise raises the demand on the body for carnitine. Additionally, carnitine supplements have been shown to increase muscle function and offer greater resistance to fatigue. Blood fats are more efficiently oxidized, too.

Naturally, the sports world has become fascinated with carnitine. Brian Leibovitz, one of the pioneer investigators of this nutrient, requested that Bill Toomey, the 1968 decathlon champion, add carnitine to his diet. Toomey, then 44 years old, did. Within three weeks the athlete lost weight, dropping from 215 to 200 pounds, and he reported that his squat and bench weights rose by more than 20 pounds.

There may be possibilities for carnitine beyond encouraging weight loss and upping strength. Carnitine appears to help the heart as well as contribute to weight loss. When naturally synthesized carnitine is bolstered by 400 milligrams of carnitine taken three times a day, blood triglyceride levels are reduced. This is accomplished by increasing the proper metabolism of fats to energy. Some people lose blood triglycerides with daily supplementation of just 500 milligrams of carnitine; others need the full 1200 milligrams mentioned above.

Biochemists at Sports Research, Inc., in Houston have warned me against using the synthetic forms of this nutrient: D-carnitine or DL-carnitine. "We produce just L-carnitine because that's the only effective and harmless form," Dr. Luke Bucci told me. "Patients using DL-carnitine have developed neurological symptoms. Side effects are equally damaging from D-carnitine. Feedback to our product relative to weight loss is excellent."

A frequently asked question is how carnitine speeds the burning of fat in cells. Researchers I.B. Fritz, of the University of Michigan, and K.T.N Yue, after many years of investigation, discovered the answer.

Our trillions of cells have mitochondria, miniscule furnaces in which fats and carbohydrates are changed into energy. Fat has difficulty penetrating the inner sanctum of the mitochondria, where the action is, but carnitine and an enzyme at the inner mitochondria wall join hands with fat and move it into the mitochondria for burning. A low level of body carnitine means that the delivery of fat into the mitochondria will be slow, leaving surplus fat to accumulate.

Strict vegetarians could end up low in carnitine, as in vitamin B-12, because neither vegetables nor fruit have more than a negligible amount of lysine or carnitine. Inability to synthesize carnitine is an exceptional genetic flaw that brings on a rare kind of muscular dystrophy whose major symptom is incredible muscle weakness. Carnitine supplementation often produces dramatic reversal of this condition.

In instances of high accumulation of fatty acids and triglycerides in the bloodstream, researchers in this field believe, it might be well for physicians to suspect at least partial carnitine deficiency. Without the carnitine to make the mitochondrial transport system efficient, fats and triglycerides can't penetrate properly to be burned. What else can these fats do but continue to make the rounds of the circulatory system?

It is not generally known that suboptimal carnitine status can cause a multitude of cardiovascular complications and at the same time block weight loss.

Many preventive medicine specialists recommend taking an L-carnitine supplement rather than adding a great deal of meat to the diet, although carnitine supplementation is not inexpensive. Sometimes a liver defect can prevent the synthesizing of carnitine from lysine, in which case carnitine supplementation may be advisable.

With the cholesterolphobia craze, some individuals have virtually cut meat from their diet and have deprived themselves of carnitine—a means of combatting heart and artery problems and increasing weight loss. Folk remedy restoratives rich in carnitine are beef bouillon and chicken soup in the United States and beef tea in Scotland.

It has been found that carnitine functions in the mitochondria much as thyroid hormone does in metabolism: like a carburetor.

An exciting experiment was conducted at the American McGaw company to demonstrate the fat-burning ability of carnitine. Fatty livers were encouraged to develop in laboratory animals. When the animals were fed carnitine supplements, their liver fat began to disappear. The speed at which the fat dissipated was in direct proportion to how much carnitine was administered.

One of the most dramatic discoveries about carnitine was that it is helpful in reducing fat depots in various parts of the human anatomy.

No matter from which angle the subject of carnitine in the human body is studied, it seems that its value continues to be verified. In experiments at the University of British Columbia, biochemists discovered that mice that are genetically prone to be obese have almost 50 percent less carnitine than do mice that are genetically prone to remain lean.

Carnitine appears to have great promise. Numerous laboratories throughout the world are involved in double-blind studies to determine whether or not the glowing results from experiments can be duplicated. Many knowledge gaps still exist about this nutrient.

How are preventive medicine specialists reacting to use of carnitine for patients? Results have been promising for those with whom I have checked. Thus far, most of the doctors seem to combine carnitine therapy with reduced dietary calories and a vigorous exercise regimen.

In chapter 11, "How to Beat the Stubborn Setpoint," I touched briefly upon evening primrose oil and its effectiveness in bringing about weight loss in individuals who were more than 10 percent above normal weight. This product didn't work with normal-weights or the slightly overweight.

A special capability of evening primrose oil emerged from a weight loss experiment conducted in the Metabolic Unit of the University of Wales. Ten super-obese patients—at least 40 percent above ideal weight—who were unable to reduce further on a 1000 calorie diet were given six evening primrose oil capsules a day with their usual diet. They resumed weight loss again: 4.8 kilograms (about 10.5 pounds) at the end of six weeks.

Then, too, sodium in the patients' red blood cells dropped

significantly, revealing starkly that evening primrose oil had sparked this high-energy-burning enzyme system in cells in all parts of the body.

A further dramatic finding came from this study. Brown fat activity of some patients was observed through the capability of thermography. Evening primrose oil had evidently expanded the area of active brown fat. This did not happen in control subjects who were given diet only.

Another laboratory experiment—this with genetically obese mice—demonstrated that evening primrose oil puts the brakes on gaining weight. This, researchers feel, hints that it may be helpful to human beings with flaws in metabolism. In cases such as these, evening primrose oil can limit weight gain and even promote weight loss. Nevertheless, David Horrobin, Ph.D., one of the world's foremost authorities on evening primrose oil, finds that it will probably not work if obesity results from overeating only.

The exciting part of evening primrose oil is that as a fore-runner to prostaglandins, it can make numerous contributions to health and well-being over and above enhancing the possibilities of losing weight. Like carnitine and other products mentioned earlier, this is a multiphase food supplement with the most glowing possibilities, many of which have not as yet been fully investigated.

CHAPTER TWENTY-THREE

HERBAL WAIST DISPOSAL

And God said, Behold I have given you every herb bearing seed, which is upon the face of all the earth . . . Genesis 1:29 (KJV)

SOMETIMES those stubborn surplus pounds appear to have a will of their own—an iron will. Then your best efforts to win seem none too good. However, rather than quit, try something new.

That "something new" could be herbs to reduce your hips, slim you down amidships, and melt your thighs down to size.

To paraphrase the scripture above, God has given you and me every herb bearing seed on the face of the earth. (As a matter of fact, herbs are mentioned more than three thousand times in the Bible, so they definitely belong in a book called *The Diet Bible*.

With tens of thousands of herbs, how do you choose the right ones? Folk medicine through the ages has helped isolate those that are effective.

Eleven herbs are said to contribute to losing weight. Some people use individual ones on the list that follows. Others use them all. Here they are with a brief description.

Chickweed. This low-growing plant of the pink family, found as a weed in lawns and gardens, has been used as a green and as a poultice for centuries. Chickweed has been discovered to contribute to the breaking-down of fat in the body.

Licorice Root. A European perennial plant of the legume family, the licorice root has blue spike-shaped flowers and short, flat pods. The dried root of the plant or the black syrup from it is used as medicine or as a main ingredient in candy.

As an herb, licorice root is food for the adrenal glands. It is supposedly necessary to eat a meal at least every five hours, that is, if you want to lose weight. After five hours you begin to run on your adrenals rather than burn body fat. This harms the body and frustrates weight loss. Licorice root also contributes to keeping the blood sugar level up for energy.

Safflower. This is a yellow, thistlelike annual plant that has large, orange flower heads and seeds from which oils for foods, medicines, and paints are derived. Safflower contributes to neutralizing uric acid. People who have been on diets or fasts experience a buildup of uric acid. The uric acid level was raised in the first place because of poor diet, which contributed to overweight.

Gotu Kola. An herb noted for contributing to energy for body and brain, Gotu Kola is a natural stimulant that revives fasters and dieters who have become physically lethargic and mentally sluggish.

Mandrake. A nightshade plant found in the Mediterranean regions, the mandrake has a short stem, purple or white flowers, and a thick root that some botanists think is shaped in the form of the human body. The root has been used for medicine for ages. It is said to feed and cleanse the liver (an efficiently functioning liver is essential to weight loss). Mandrake serves as a mild laxative. Constipated individuals usually have weight problems.

Echinecea. This is an herb that seems to possess unusual powers of coping with bacteria, in much the same way as penicillin acts. Such a function is necessary when individuals fast or go on a low-calorie diet, because poison waste circulates through the body on its way to removal. Unlike penicillin, echinecea brings no ill effects to those taking it.

Black Walnut. A rich source of iodine, black walnut makes an important contribution to supplying this major food of the thyroid gland—essential to forceful heartbeat and delivery of oxygen and nutrients to all body cells, efficient carrying off of wastes, and full liver function. It is said to kill microorganisms that give off waste material toxic to the body.

Fennel. A tall herb of the parsley family, fennel has yellow flowers whose aromatic seeds are used in cooking and in medicines. This herb serves dieters in two ways: curbing appetite, and relieving accumulated gas brought on by dietary changes for weight reduction.

Hawthorne. This is a thorny shrub or small tree of the rose family with white, pink, or red flowers and red fruits resembling mini-apples. Hawthorne is an all-purpose herb. Supposedly, it strengthens the heart, which is usually under strain when a person is markedly overweight. Strengthening of the heart is important to enable it to take the added stress of dieting. The oldest known herb for the heart, hawthorne has been used to manage edema, or waterlogged tissues.

Dandelion. Everyone who has ever cared for a lawn, particularly in the north temperate zone, is familiar with this unwelcome guest, an herb with jagged, green leaves and a yellow flower. Used as a food, for salad greens, and as a basis for wine, the dandelion is said to feed and cleanse the liver. If the liver is toxic and underfunctioning, it is virtually impossible to lose weight. Dandelion is also a natural diuretic, helping the body throw off fluids and thus contributing to weight loss.

Papaya. This cannot accurately be categorized as an herb. It is definitely a fruit from a tropical American tree resembling a palm. The oblong yellow-green fruit has one of the highest enzyme contents of any fruit anywhere.

During dieting much waste is thrown off from the body. Along with this waste some friendly bacteria are also evacuated. Papaya, with the other herbs mentioned, encourages the restoration of these friendly bacteria lost by the body.

Additionally, papaya's enzymes make for better digestion, important for deriving full nutrient values from foods and helping to ensure that undigested molecules do not escape into the bloodstream and bring on food allergies. Allergies are notorious for contributing to weight gain or retention.

People taking all the above herbs with their usual diet discover after ten days to two weeks that they visit the bathroom a few more times than usual. Material passed should not be confused with runny stool; it is only the removal of excess waste material. At the end of this period, when all excess waste is gone, the bowel movement will again be normal. Those most familiar with this regimen say that normal elimination is a bowel movement after every normal-size meal. Anything less than one bowel movement per day is regarded as constipation.

The "Combination" regimen appears to have promise.

CHAPTER TWENTY-FOUR

THOSE BEAUTIFUL BIBLE FOODS

We remember the fish which we did eat in Egypt freely; the cucumbers, and the melons, and the leeks, and the onions, and the garlick.'' Numbers 11:5 (KJV)

*O*UTSIDE of science fiction there's no time machine to propel us back to biblical days, when it was easier to stay thin and well nourished for these three reasons:

1. People lived far more physically active lives next to nature.
2. Foods were grown according to God's laws.
3. Foods were eaten in ways to preserve the most nutrients.

This connectedness with God disappeared subtly and gradually with the evolution of civilization: the rise of cities, the distancing of man from his food supply, mechanization, and, now, incessant advertising in the mass media. Yet, there is an easy way to recapture connectedness with biblical times and foods, most of which are still available, and to use them to lose weight naturally.

As the opening Scripture indicates, the foods the Israelites missed most after escaping from Egypt with the miraculous parting of the Red Sea were fish, vegetables, and fruits.

The Egyptians supplied the ocean catch of the day as well as freshwater relatives of the sun bass family that were raised in numerous ponds with water from the Nile river. These fish were roasted on hot embers or boiled in water or oil. What could not be eaten at the time was sun-dried (an excellent way to preserve most of the nutrients) or salted and sun-dried (not as healthful a method).

However, the Israelites favored broiling fish right on the embers, as verified in two places in the Scriptures: Luke 24:42 and John 21:9. As a matter of fact, broiling in this fashion is the only method of cooking fish mentioned in the Bible.

The best illustration that broiling was the preferred method of fish preparation is a work of art in the Gizeh Museum of Egypt, in Cairo, showing shepherds broiling fish on the fire and then wiping off the ashes with tiny bundles of straw.

For the common people of Israel fish was far more important than meat, because they could afford it daily. Meat was a luxury item reserved for special celebrations or for the middle class and the wealthy, who showed their status by serving meat—often several kinds—just as today's materially successful person sports a Rolls Royce, Mercedes, Jaguar, or Maserati.

Two passages of the New Testament involving Jesus illustrate that fish and bread were the main daily fare for the common people. In Luke 11:11 Jesus asks: "If a son shall ask bread of any of you that is a father, will he give him a stone? Or if he ask a fish, will he for a fish give him a serpent?"

In John 6, we read about the miracles of the loaves and fishes. There were five thousand to be fed, and a perplexed disciple, Andrew, told Jesus: "There is a lad here, which hath five barley loaves and two small fishes: but what are they among so many?" (John 6:9)

Then Jesus told the men to sit down on the grass. "And Jesus took the loaves; and when he had given thanks, he distributed to the disciples, and the disciples to them that were set down; and likewise of the fishes as much as they would." (John: 6:11)

And typical of the frugality of that day's common person, Jesus ordered his disciples to gather up the fragments that remained, that nothing be lost. "Therefore, they gathered them together and filled twelve baskets with the fragments of the five barley loaves, which remained over and above unto them that had eaten." (John 6:13)

The sources of fresh fish? The Sea of Galilee and the Mediterranean. In Zephaniah 1:10 we read about the fish gate in Jerusalem, where sun-dried or salted fish imported by Tyrian dealers were also sold. Cured fish, one of the major export items from Egypt, moved fast until the Israelites learned the curing process and established a curing place at the south end of the Sea of Galilee. Many a meal that Jesus ate featured fish as its main course.

Another reason fish was more popular than meat was that meat did not lend itself as readily as fish to preservation, and for this reason it was hard to justify killing an animal far larger in unit size than a fish unless it was a religious holiday, such as the yearly pilgrimage to the sanctuary (Haggim), a time of guests, a family feast, a wedding, a circumcision ceremony, or a bar mitzvah. The prodigal son's return was the occasion for preparing the fatted calf. (Luke 15:23)

Of course, superrich King Solomon, the man who had everything before Nieman Marcus did, was not restricted in meat supply. Each day he and his court enjoyed "ten fat oxen, twenty pasture-fed cattle, a hundred sheep, besides harts [deer] gazelles, roebucks [male of the roe deer] and fatted fowl." (I Kings 4:23)

A second reason animals were slaughtered reluctantly or only for special occasions was because some of them were used for other purposes, for example, as a source of wool or of milk. Other food products could be made from milk.

Because the Passover lamb was required to be roasted, roasting was the most popular method of cooking small to large animals. This was done customarily on a fire made from wood of a vine. Several historical sources state that roasting was the only method of preparing meat until the Jews returned to Palestine from Egypt and learned from the Canaanites how to boil meat in water or in oil.

Pottage—a thick soup or stew—was also popular. It was usually made from lentils, garlic, and onions, although the Israelites were creative in blending any permitted meat, such as mutton or lamb, with lentils or beans.

The mess of pottage for which Esau sold his birthright is indeed a savory concoction of lentils cooked with meat and onions and seasoned with garlic and herbs. Sometimes suet was added for extra flavor. *The Diet Bible* recipes in the next chapter will offer some tasty, low-calorie pottages. Why was this dish called by such an inelegant name? Simply because it was eaten right out of the pot in which it was cooked.

In Ezekiel 24:3–5 we find an excellent recipe for a lamb stew, rich in bone marrow:

"Set on a pot, set it on, and also pour water into it: Gather the pieces thereof into it, even every good piece, the thigh and the shoulder; fill it with choice bones. Take the choice of the flock, and burn also the bones under it, and make it boil well, and let them seethe the bones of it therein."

Lamb was the most common animal eaten by the poor and the rich, particularly when guests were present. After festive occasions the poor were especially pleased, because they could sell the lamb fleece for extra income. Because slaughtering animals and preparing them for cooking was an arduous and unpleasant task, the men of the house handled these activities and were even responsible for roasting or boiling the meat.

Chicken were known in Israel in Old and New Testament times, but hard to get. However, pigeons and turtledoves were numerous, cheap, and popular with poor as well as moderate income people.

Although meat was scarce in biblical times, grains were usually plentiful: bulgar wheat, barley, and corn. When crops of wheat and barley were poor, millet and spelt (fitches), mentioned in the King James version, were used as cereals and in bread.

It was not uncommon to eat fresh kernels of barley, millet, and wheat right from the fields. Mentioned many times in the Bible, "parched corn," a term for any parched grain, was made by heating almost ripe wheat on an iron griddle or on something similar to today's frying pan. Parched grain, a favorite food for laborers, could be eaten as is or made into meal or flour.

A crude way of grinding barley, corn, or wheat was to crush it with a pestle. Bruised grain could be eaten without further preparation. It could be used as porridge, too. Grains, as well as lentils or beans, were cooked in water or olive oil with onions, leeks, and garlic, or in butter and, when available, with meat or fish.

An alternative way of preparing grain was by grinding it

with a stone handmill called a quern. Mixed with water or milk, flour was made into a batter. Unleavened bread was made from batter used at once and served at the sacred Passover meal. To make leavened bread or cakes, the batter was allowed to stand and collect yeast from the air, or it was treated with stored yeast or leaven for baking or for carrying by travelers to be baked as needed. For ceremonial purposes or for rare dessert treats such as date or fig cakes, flour was ground particularly fine.

When we talk about "our daily bread," that is the correct name for it. In biblical times, people ate bread at every meal, mainly barley bread for the poor and wheat bread for the wealthy. The latter was usually made from bulgar wheat or sometimes from emmer, a primitive form of wheat.

Women of the house had to take special measures to make the heavy barley bread dough rise: using strong millet and barley yeast. Bread was formed to come out in a round shape, which is the basis for the biblical expression, "a round of bread." Baked right on hot embers in the small household oven, this low-slung loaf was made to be torn off, not cut.

Most of the baking and cooking fell to the woman of the house: grinding meal, preparing batter, baking bread and cakes, and making butter and cheese. Surprisingly, even some women in the royal family were called upon to perform these household tasks.

Over and above grains and the products made from them was another staple: milk. There are at least nineteen Bible references to Palestine as the "land of milk and honey," but the milk referred to is that from goats or from sheep, the second choice.

Few cows existed in the land because of the poor pasturage and because milk from other animals was much preferred. Camel's milk was drunk by Old Testament people, but it was usually shunned in the New Testament because it sours more quickly than other milks in desert heat and takes some palate adjustments for first-timers.

The butter derived from cream ranged from a heavy, soured product to the semisolid that we know as butter. It was made from heavy cream that was deposited into a big skin bag suspended by three sticks and vigorously shaken until the cream solidified. The butter referred to in Genesis 18:8 appears to have been a thick, sour milk called *laban*, a semifluid similar to yogurt or kefir.

The cheese mentioned in I Kings 17:18—Jesse sent a gift of it to the captain in charge of the troops to which his sons were attached—appears to have been *laban*, not cheese as we know it today. However, the Israelites did have cheese like ours. They drained the fluid from curdled milk and then salted the curd and molded it into hand-sized lumps, which they left in the sun to dry.

In this land of "milk and honey," it is appropriate to say, all Palestine honey wasn't really honey, honey! In some instances it was thickened grape juice or the gooey, sugary sap pressed out of dates.

Of course, the Israelites had the real thing, too, found where wild bees had deposited it in hollows of rocks or trees. They found so much of it that they exported some to Tyre. The Israelites knew about bee culture but never had to adopt it given their honey's natural abundance.

Honey served as refined white sugar does today and was also used for medicinal purposes. Fine pastries for special occasions were made with honey, which was also mixed into drinks such as milk, added to certain fish, and even eaten straight. Proverbs 25:16 warns about overdoing the honey routine: "Hast thou found honey? Eat so much as is sufficient for thee, lest thou be filled therewith, and vomit it."

Not on a level with honey but a much more substantial food, eggs began growing in popularity in New Testament times. They had always been desirable in Old Testament days but were rarely available then because the source, wild birds, was sporadic and undependable. Then, when geese were introduced from Egypt and domestic fowl from India, the supply began to catch up with demand.

Roman soldiers are said to have been egg-happy and to have brought in dozens of different recipes for preparing eggs. Before them, the Egyptians had exported simple spoons of bone or terra cotta, certain ones with pointed ends were designed for eating boiled eggs and shellfish.

Neither eggs nor any food in Palestine had the versatility of the olive in the economy of the Israelites. Its oil was used for religious and healing purposes; for anointing; for burning in lamps to illuminate; for spreading on bread like butter; and for cooking. The olive itself was also edible.

Thirty passages in the Bible mention it, some extolling the olive's many virtues. Palestine had so many olive trees, which thrived in the land, that it was able to export much olive oil to neighboring countries.

Another of Palestine's key fruits, the grape, was pressed into wine mainly, but the best of the crop was sun-dried to make raisins, which were eaten as is or used in making pastries or formed and compressed into cakes. In I Samuel 25:18, Abigail brings a hundred such raisin cakes to David. Along with figs and dates, raisins served as a compact food to be taken on journeys by travelers.

Figs were eaten fresh, sun-dried, or pressed into round or square cakes. Fig cakes and barley bread were usually the staples for poor travelers in the Middle-East. Israelite cakes of figs were even sold as far away as Rome.

In one instance a fig cake was used as a compress that caused the dying King Hezekiah to be healed: "And Isaiah said, Take a lump of figs. And they took and laid it on the boil, and he recovered." (2 Kings 20:7)

Like figs dates were one of the favorite fruits of the Israelites, particularly succulent, extra-sweet dates from Jericho. A date honey called *dibs* was made by boiling the fruit almost to a liquid.

While information about most fruits in the Bible is straightforward and uncontested, that about the apple seems to cause an endless difference of opinion among experts on the Scriptures. Most authorities say that the apples mentioned in Old Testament were not really apples but actually quinces or citrons. These experts refer to an apple tree victimized in a locust plague (Joel 1:12) and the dialogue in the Song of Solomon (2:5), in which a loved one asks for refreshment with apples. No one, however, seems to touch Adam and Eve's apple in the Garden of Eden.

The argument is that the apples referred to can't be apples as we know them because most apple trees can only rarely grow in Palestine, to which they are not native. One authority claims to have seen an apple tree growing luxuriantly. Another expert says this expert was mistaken. On the basis of philology, still another authority refers to the word *tappuah*, Hebrew for apple, but he's shot down because of the fact that apple trees were scarce in Palestine.

Various Bible texts refer to a shady tree with fragrant, pleasant-tasting golden fruit that was the symbol of love, and biblical scholars insist that this is the quince, which grows widely in the Holy Land, or the apricot or persimmon.

Far more popular than the apple or the quince to Old and New Testament people were two kinds of melons: the watermelon and the flesh melon (similar to the cantaloupe), both refreshing, low-calorie, and filling foods.

A favorite fruit of the people of the Bible was the rich, red pomegranate. Noted for its sour juice, it was used in much the same way we use lemons—as a favorite ingredient in sherbet.

Mulberries, too, were frequently eaten by the Old and New Testament people. In His parable on faith in Luke 17:6, Jesus refers to the mulberry tree by its then-name: sycamine.

About the only thing husks have in common with the mulberry is that they both grow on trees. Husks are long, flat, leathery brown pods with sweet pulp. A vastly underrated food in the Bible's prodigal son story, husks grow on what we call carob trees, which were common in near-eastern countries, including Palestine, in Bible times. These husks were usually fed to cattle.

And the prodigal son felt abused eating cattle fodder to keep alive—he could have done a lot worse nutritionally! Carob has a host of nicknames: St. Johns bread, egyptian fig, and honey locust. The term "honey locust" leads a few Bible scholars to believe that the "locusts" of the "locusts and honey" on which John the Baptist survived were not one of the 800 edible varieties of locusts (migratory grasshoppers) but the honey locust, or carob, pods.

Yet carob, now mainly used as a healthful chocolate substitute, is rich in carbohydrates (about 70 percent), vitamins A, B (three members of the B family), and D, and many minerals, the most prominent of which are calcium (carob contains three times as much calcium as an equivalent amount of milk), iron, and magnesium. Carob contains fewer calories and less fat and sodium per pound than chocolate, requires less sweetening than chocolate to make it taste good, and includes no oxalic acid (which chocolate has), which links with calcium and draws it out of the body.

Only three of today's nuts get even a moderate play in the Bible: walnuts, almonds, and pistachios. Many walnut trees dotted the Palestinian landscape, and the nuts were eaten right out of the shell and sometimes added to sweet fruit. Likewise, almonds grew wild on Mount Carmel and in Moab. They were blended with dates or figs as a dessert; and the Medes mixed them in bread dough for variety. Pistachios carefully split open and roasted made a tasty snack and an addition to date and fig dishes.

Above all kinds of food—nuts, flesh, fruits, and vegetables—the Israelites had the greatest longing for fish and, following that, cucumbers when they escaped from Egypt after the miraculous parting of the Red Sea, as witnessed by the passage from Numbers 11:5 quoted at the beginning of the chapter.

Two major species of cucumbers excited the appetites of the Israelites with a passion hard for us to conceive. These alluring, green vegetables tasted cool and refreshing in the desert heat and were eaten in one of several ways: right from the garden with the green skin on (remember, no harmful pesticides, herbicides or fungicides then existed); in slices dipped in *laban* (the yogurt-like form of soured milk); dipped in vinegar and eaten with barley or wheat bread; stuffed with mincemeat and various spices; and pressed into juice for drinking.

The Israelites so prized their cucumbers that they posted watchmen around the vast cucumber fields to frighten away the jackals, wild dogs that roamed in packs, that stealthily invaded the grounds to feast on their favorite vegetables.

After leaving Egypt the Israelites also longed for leeks, onions, and garlic. The leek is an onionlike vegetable with a small bulb and a cylindrical stem that was eaten raw with fragments of bread, sliced and left bathed in vinegar for an intermingling of flavors, or liberally added to pottage.

Onions, leeks, scallions, and garlic are all members of the lily family. They are not as lovely to look at as lilies, but their distinctively pungent odors and flavors make them a worthy addition to pottage, other stews, or cooked eggs. Slaves who built the pyramids of Egypt were given a daily ration of onions and garlic, both of which were said to boost their strength and endurance (and most certainly have added strength to their breath). Both Egyptians and Israelites ate onions and garlic straight, often with fragments of barley bread. Oh, to have had the Israel-Egypt monopoly on breath mints!

Way back in 3758 B.C. Egyptian slaves on the construction site of the great pyramid of Cheops went on strike—they sat down and refused to work—because their taskmasters had cut out their daily ration of garlic. Good news! They got their garlic, and their taskmasters got their pyramid! Ancient Vikings and Phoenician seamen insisted on having a big load of garlic in the hold before going aboard for a long voyage. They were the first ancient mariners who lived by the slogan "Don't leave home without it!"

The curative and preventive medical powers of onions and garlic are legendary, and, for garlic, particularly well documented. Over the past 5000 years garlic has been the single most effective folk remedy, with a record for doing amazing things:

1. Serving as a natural antibiotic, killing microorganisms that cause colds, flu, pneumonia, and tuberculosis.
2. Correcting intestinal disorders: gas, infection, and worms.
3. Purging body pollutants.
4. Clearing up dysentery and diarrhea.
5. Reducing elevated blood pressure.
6. Lowering high blood cholesterol levels.
7. Improving circulation of patients with atherosclerosis.
8. Keeping blood platelets slippery so that clots don't form accidentally and block circulation.

A Russian scientist conducted experiments that showed that all of garlic's power isn't in its odor. Researcher T.D. Yanovich put several wriggly bacteria colonies into garlic juice. Three minutes later they stopped moving. Next he added garlic juice to a culture of bacteria. Immediately, the bacteria quickly shifted away from the garlic juice, and two minutes later, some of the microorganisms stopped moving. Ten minutes later there was no movement at all.

Some years ago the respected English medical journal *Lancet* presented an article about quick cures of the most stubborn kinds of tuberculosis and pneumonia. At the time these ailments killed more patients than any other diseases.

W. C. Minchin, M.D., who headed the tuberculosis ward at Dublin's Kells Hospital, had so much faith in garlic therapy that he invited other physicians to send him their obstinate cases, some of whom were only a few thousand gasps from death.

Dr. Minchin worked to overwhelm negative conditions with garlic. He had patients swallow garlic or its juice several times a day, inhale garlic fumes many times daily, and hold still for garlic compresses on their chest or whatever the infected part was: skin, bones, or joints.

His success was phenomenal. One of many spectacular cases stands out: A ten-year old boy was referred to him for amputation of a hand whose bones were being eaten away by tuberculosis. The doctor applied fresh garlic compresses to the hand daily, and after six weeks the condition was healed!

Although deodorized garlic juice and capsules under the brand name Kyolic can be bought in health food stores everywhere, no one has as yet figured out how to make fresh garlic a little more socially acceptable.

I take liquid garlic daily, and I'm a fanatic about using fresh garlic in just about everything—meat, fish, soups, stews—everything but homemade ice cream. What excitement raw garlic adds to ordinary dishes such as pottage while also building up the health of eaters! If you're taking garlic just for the health of it, the deodorized form seems most advantageous. However, if you insist on raw garlic, well . . . you may not win popularity contests, but you will always be assured a seat on a crowded bus.

Now, beyond onions and garlic are the following herbs, which the Israelites found indispensible and which seem worthy of brief comment:

Capers. This prickly, trailing Mediterranean bush produces tiny green flower buds, which were pickled and used to flavor sauces and major dishes.

Cassia. Inasmuch as this condiment was referred to in the Bible as "scented cassia," many authorities think it was probably cinnamon, which, as it was then, is used mainly in desserts.

Coriander. Dried seeds from this member of the carrot family contain an aromatic oil that gives flavoring to food or medicines. It is used as a seasoning, like caraway seed and cumin.

Cumin. A member of the carrot family, this herb has aromatic seedlike fruit similar to the caraway seed, a relative. The seeds were used as a seasoning for food and in medicines.

Dill. A member of the carrot family, this plant has pungent and aromatic seeds that impart a unique flavoring to soups, stews, gravies, salads, and pickles.

Mint. An aromatic herb, the mint is noted for cool flavoring and the volatile, fragrant perfume given off by its leaves and stems.

Mustard. This plant is distinguished by attractive yellow flowers with slender pods containing round seeds, which are dried, reduced to powder, and then moistened with fluid to form a seasoning that imparts a pungent almost stinging flavor to foods.

Rosemary. This is an evergreen plant of the mint family whose light blue flowers and leaves give off a fragrant minty oil used to enhance food flavors.

Rue. The foliage, fruit, and flowers of this woody shrub or miniature tree give off an aromatic flavoring and fragrance for foods, perfumes, and medicines.

Saffron. This member of the iris family is characterized by funnel-shaped purple flowers featuring orange stigmas. The stigmas have a strong, aromatic perfume and flavoring, which are used in many kinds of dishes.

This brief roundup of Old and New Testament foods and flavorings will serve as an introduction to the *Bible Diet* menu and related dishes in the next chapter.

Why were the Israelites generally of moderate weight? There are three obvious clues, two historical and one based on modern biochemistry: 1) They used up calories like mad with a super-active physical life; 2) They were undereaters or average eaters; and 3) their choice of meats—sheep and lamb—are the richest discovered to date in carnitine, the nutrient that makes the brown fat burn hottest. Sheep muscle meat contains 210 mg of carnitine per 100 grams of edible content. Lamb muscle meat rates second-highest at 78 mg per 100 grams. Next comes beef, with 64. Then there's a dramatic dropoff of nine times to chicken muscle, with just 7.5

It is true that the poor people were only infrequent meat eaters. However, they ate fish—another high rater in carnitine content—almost daily.

Middle- and upper-class Israelites ate meat much more regularly, along with a great deal of fish. When they did, they stoked the biochemical furnace high and burned off the fat with carnitine.

The next chapter features many menus with carnitine-rich foods—lamb, sheep, beef, fish, and chicken. Inasmuch as we eat far more meat than the Israelites did, many of the *Diet Bible* weight loss recipes that follow contain lamb and other foods with carnitine to help us control weight.

Bon appetit!

CHAPTER TWENTY-FIVE

THE DIET BIBLE DIET

Before Beginning

*I*N a sense, this introduction is like the book of Genesis in the Bible. It deals with creation—in this instance, the creation for both women and men of an individual 30-Day weight-control program unlike any other in content, in ease of preparation, and in effectiveness.

What's so unique about it? Many things. It provides:

1. A hearty, high-powered breakfast.
2. A rich amount of carnitine.
3. Low-fat foods.
4. Natural, nutrient-packed, organically grown foods.
5. Delightful, tasty meals that make dieting easy.
6. Quick preparation.
7. Protection against food allergens.
8. Reversal of the customary feeding pattern for greatest weight loss.

Let me elaborate.

A Hearty Breakfast

Conventional diets starve the weight-control candidate at breakfast, causing constant and acute hunger. The dieter thus suffers martyrdom all day and sooner or later violates the diet.

The Diet Bible diet provides a daily, stick-to-the-ribs breakfast that elevates the morning blood sugar and keeps it level to lunchtime, making it far easier for the dieter to adhere to the rest of the day's meals. Several studies bear out this claim.

People in Bible times ate a hearty breakfast that often included fish or, when they could afford it, meat.

High Carnitine Content

Carnitine, as mentioned earlier, causes stored fat to be burned. Middle Easterners unknowingly ate carnitine-rich foods: lamb (one of the highest carnitine-content meats), beef, fish, and poultry—wild game birds in Old Testament times and later domesticated fowl, including chicken. Matthew 26:75 (KJV) confirms domesticated fowl in the new Testament, when Jesus says to Peter, ". . . Before the cock crows, thou shalt deny me thrice."

Low Fat Intake

Many Israelites obeyed the injunction in Leviticus 7:23 (KJV), "Ye shall eat no manner of fat of ox or of sheep or of goat," and therefore accumulated little body fat. As pointed out earlier, dietary fats readily become stored body fats.

This doesn't mean they didn't drink whole milk and eat laban, yogurt made from whole milk, and butter. However, they didn't consume a large amount of dairy products.

Natural, Nutrient-Packed, Organically Grown Foods

The Diet Bible diet calls for God-given, natural grains grown with respect for the soil such as meal or flour stone-ground from wheat, millet, corn, barley, and rye, and cereals or bread made from them. These foods provide vitamins and minerals in proper relationships and fiber to promote regularity, and they satisfy appetite on fewer calories than today's processed versions, protecting blood sugar from the dangerously low drops that make a person voracious for more foods. The same goes for legumes—peas and beans—and whole brown rice.

Daniel and his contemporaries in the Old Testament could be sustained on a vegetarian diet because soils then were allowed to rest periodically and were enriched with natural ferilizers. Organically grown, fresh vegetables and fruits have a better balance of vitamins and minerals and tend to turn off the appetite earlier than nonorganic, pesticide-laden produce. Health food supermarkets are regularly supplied with organic fruits and vegetables.

Delightful, Tasty Foods That Make Dieting Easy

Many conventional diets offer such unphotogenic and unpleasant foods that even a Spartan couldn't stomach long enough to lose weight. Foods featured in the Diet Bible diet look great and taste great.

Quick Preparation

The Diet Bible diet offers simple, easily and quickly prepared foods. Many conventional diets feature meals that are so difficult and tedious to prepare that the dieter soon gives up in despair. What foods cannot be bought in a supermarket can be obtained in a health food store. Every different kind of bread called for in the recipes can be bought in a health food store and frozen in plastic envelopes, one or two slices at a time, and later toasted. All muffins called for can be obtained in health food stores, too.

During the first week of the 30-day Diet Bible diet program, I offer a way of preparing a whole week's or even a month's basic menus that takes no more than two hours on an evening or weekend.

Protection Against Food Allergens

Many diets are self-defeating because they repeat foods to which dieters are sensitive or allergic. This causes water retention and weight gain. Frequent repetition of allergenic foods also aggravates sensitivities and allergies.

As insurance against such a problem, the Diet Bible diet tries not to repeat the same food more than once every five days, and it avoids multi-ingredient prepared flavorings and sauces and, when possible, recipes with many ingredients. In this way the diet minimizes the chance of sensitivities and allergies and maximizes the possibility of weight loss. Few individuals are sensitive or allergic to the sprouts used in some of the salads featured.

Reversal of the Feeding Pattern for Greatest Weight Loss

Several studies show that by eating the highest-calorie meal in the morning and then a lighter lunch and an even lighter dinner, one can lose weight dramatically without changing the total number of calories consumed. One such study reported in the *Louisiana State Medical Journal* was mentioned in an earlier chapter.

If you protest that you "can't eat breakfast," take a tip from one of my doctor friends: "Simply skip several dinners, and you'll soon be unbelievably hungry at breakfast time. It's a matter of starting and fixing a new worthwhile habit."

You may ask, "How can I possibly eat a light meal at night when I'm invited out socially or on business?" Sometimes you can't. I try to limit myself to one or two dinners out a week, and I have as many business meals as possible at breakfast time, when I can eat fairly heavily. Another alternative I use is eating small amounts of everything served in order to adhere to the diet and at the same time please my hostess or host. It can be done, and you can do it.

So much for that problem. How about the one of changing the habits of a lifetime and eating things that most of us are unaccustomed to for breakfast—fish, for instance, as they often did in Bible times, and meats. Habits of a lifetime can be changed by repetition of new eating patterns.

A high-protein breakfast from the Diet Bible diet does a whole lot more than keep your blood sugar elevated for greater consistent energy and less hunger thoughout your day. It makes the mind more alert, as shown by several studies of Dr. Richard Wurtman of MIT. Conversely, the high-carbohydrate diet—dry cereal and black coffee or just a donut or sweet roll—offers a spurt of energy and then a collapse like a leaky balloon, bringing with it drowsiness and sluggish thinking and remembering. This is hardly the physical or mental condition that vaults us to the top in this highly competitive world.

Fat of the Land

Of course, a high intake of fat undermines us, too, but for a different reason, as explained earlier. However, despite the fact that we eat less meat and fewer eggs and have switched from high- to low-fat milk, a U.S. Department of Agriculture survey reveals that our intake of fat remains unchanged.

The USDA believes that we maintain our fat intake because 60 percent of us now eat out regularly, dining on food high in hidden fats.

If you eat out, approach a restaurant as you would a mine field. Never order anything fried, only baked or broiled. And skip the gravies, sauces, and pastries. If you are famished before eating out, snack on an apple or some other fresh fruit so that you won't pig out on bread and butter.

The Diet Bible diet for women averages about 950 calories daily. The men's version averages approximately 1200 calories. Fortunately, micrometric precision in calorie counting is not as important in the Diet Bible diet as in other diets, because of the tremendous benefits in reversing eating patterns by having the heaviest meal in the morning.

In any event, you can vary the number of calories up or down to suit your own needs. As a matter of fact, some men prefer the lower calories of the women's diet and still feel well fed. To increase the number of calories, you simply eat slightly larger portions of one or more foods. To decrease the number of calories, you simply eat a bit less of one or two of the foods.

Be warned, however, that seeds and nuts are high-calorie items and one ounce more can boost your caloric intake by anywhere from 150 to 200. So, be careful.

Many of the same foods are in both the men's and women's diet. This is deliberate. Many couples—and families, for that matter—diet together. To make totally different menus for females and males would pose unbelievable logistical problems: too much unnecessary time loss in food preparation in this super-busy world, an overtaxing of refrigeration and freezing capacity, and a parade of pots and pans from here to eternity.

All right, enough of the preliminaries. Let's get to the main event!

DIET BIBLE DIET
(FOR WOMEN)
Approximately 950 Calories Daily

FIRST WEEK   TWO-HOUR COOKING THEME

This diet accents carnitine-rich foods and a meal rotation for a week's—or even a month's—eating that can be prepared in two hours on an evening or weekend.

Cook 1 cup each of millet, oats, whole-rye cereal and brown rice (this is a week's supply). Refrigerate the cooked cereals in individual, airtight plastic containers.

Prepare 1 pound of ½-inch cubes of lamb shanks and beef chuck and 1 pound of skinned chicken breast cubes, as recommended in the recipes below. Then refrigerate them in 4-ounce amounts in airtight plastic containers.

Make lentil loaf, according to the recipe below and refrigerate in 4-ounce amounts in individual airtight plastic containers.

Fix sprout salad as directed in the recipe below and refrigerate it in a large airtight plastic container. This salad can be stored without deteriorating for more than a week. All other items above can be frozen, if desired, and stored.

These instructions, and the recipes below, will be repeated in the "For Men" section in the interest of conserving your time.

FIRST WEEK TWO-HOUR COOKING THEME

Cook 2 cups of millet and refrigerate it in a sealed plastic container. Cook 1 cup each of whole-rye cereal, oats and brown rice and refrigerate them in individual plastic containers.

Prepare the following recipes:

═══ *King David's Lamb with Lentils* ═══

1 pound lamb shank	Dash cayenne
Garlic	2½ cups dried lentils
3 tablespoons olive oil	¼ cup chopped parsley
1 onion, minced	4 leeks, minced
½ teaspoon rosemary	

Cut lamb into ½-inch cubes. Insert a garlic sliver into each cube and brown them in 2 tablespoons oil; then add ½ cup water and simmer, turning cubes often and adding more water, if necessary, until meat is tender.

Saute onion in 1 tablespoon oil until translucent. Add rosemary and cayenne and bring to a boil. Add washed and strained lentils and 3 cups water. Return to boil, cover and simmer 45 minutes to 1 hour. Stir parsley and scallions into cooked lentils. Divide lentil mixture into 4 servings and top them with equal amounts of lamb cubes. Refrigerate each serving in a plastic container until ready to serve.

Bible Beef

1 pound lean chuck
1 medium-sized onion
   clove garlic

½ teaspoon marjoram
¼ teaspoon sea salt

Place 1 pound chuck cut into ½-inch cubes in frying pan. Sprinkle with marjoram and sea salt. Add 1 cup water to cover bottom of pan. Dice onions and garlic and add to chuck. Simmer, stirring often and adding water as necessary, until tender. Refrigerate ¼-pound servings in individual sealed plastic containers and refrigerate until required for rewarming.

Chicken and Leeks

1 pound boned and
   skinned chicken breasts
¼ pound leeks

¼ teaspoon sea salt
   Dash paprika

Cut chicken into ½-inch cubes and place in frying pan. Add salt, paprika and chopped leeks to chicken and cover bottom of pan with ¼-inch spring water.

Stew chicken, turning often and adding water if necessary. When tender, refrigerate in sealed plastic container.

Lentil Loaf

2 cups lentils	1 clove garlic, crushed
1 teaspoon sea salt	2 medium peeled, seeded
2 tablespoons olive oil	and chopped tomatoes
1 medium onion, minced	2 eggs, beaten

Cook lentils in 4-½ cups water with salt for 35 minutes or until done. Heat oven to 350°F.

Heat olive oil and saute onion until transparent. Add onion and oil to cooked lentils. Add all other ingredients. Add lentil mixture to oiled loaf pan, pat with fork to shape well, and bake for 45 minutes. Good hot or cold.

Refrigerate in airtight containers until ready for use.

Sprout Salad

This salad is virtually nonallergenic and can be repeated. Stored in an airtight, sealed container, sprout salad keeps for more than a week without deteriorating, as I have learned. Here is the recipe:

2 pounds bean sprouts	2 bunches seedless red or
2 red apples	green grapes
1 cup seedless raisins	1 stalk celery
1 dozen green onions	1 pound pine nuts or
	walnuts
	2 bunches cilantro

Cut apples, onions, celery and cilantro into fragments. Good with or without dressing.

FIRST THEME WEEK DIET

════════ *Day 1   Monday* ════════

Breakfast

4 ounces cooked lamb shank cubes with lentils, heated
1 cup fresh carrot juice or three small scrubbed carrots
Slice of whole grain wheat toast, lightly buttered
Glass of whole milk

Snack

1 large winesap apple

Lunch

Slice of lentil loaf, warmed
Sprout salad (all you wish) with choice of dressing
Sparkling mineral water

Snack

1 banana, medium size

Dinner

Cup of fresh cucumber and celery juice
1 cup cold, cooked millet flavored with ¼ cup unsweetened pine-
    apple juice
Camomile tea
(This high-carbohydrate meal may promote sound sleep.)

Day 2   Tuesday

Breakfast

4 ounces beef stew on base of cooked rye cereal
Sprout salad with dressing different from yesterday's
Large, baked Irish potato with a dollop of sour cream, a sprinkling
    of chives and a hint of sea salt.
Coffee substitue such as Cafix or Pero, available at health food
    stores

Snack

10 fresh strawberries in season or same amount unsweetened,
    fresh frozen

Lunch

1 hard-boiled egg
Slice of whole-rye toast
5 green olives
3 fresh plums
Sparkling mineral water

Snack

1 ounce sunflower seeds

Dinner

Bowl of warmed brown rice, lightly buttered, spread with unfil-
    tered, unprocessed honey and snowed over with cinnamon
Red Zinger tea

Day 3   Wednesday

Breakfast

1 cup warmed, diced chicken (4 ounces) and leeks served on bed
of cooked oats with dash of olive oil, if desired.
Slice of barley bread toast, lightly buttered
6 dates
Herbal tea

Snack

½ cup blueberries in season or same amount of unsweetened
frozen

Lunch

Sprout salad (all you can eat) with a dressing different from previous day's
Large, baked sweet potato, lightly buttered
¼ cup raisins
Sparkling mineral water

Snack

1 ounce pumpkin seeds

Dinner

½ medium-size, fresh cantaloupe or the same amount of fresh,
frozen melon balls.
Herbal tea

Day 4   Thursday

Breakfast

4 ounces salmon steak, broiled, garnished with capers
1 cup cooked millet, lightly buttered
Dish of cooked zucchini squash, lightly buttered
½ pink grapefruit
coffee substitute (such as Cafix or Pero, available in health food
    stores)

Snack

1 ounce pecans
Glass of soy milk

Lunch

Sprout salad (all you can eat) with vinaigrette dressing
½ cup cooked yellow corn
1 large orange
Sparkling mineral water

Dinner

½ cup raw green peas
Bowl of amaranth cereal with unsweetened cherry juice
Herbal tea

Day 5   Friday

Repeat Monday

Day 6   Saturday

Repeat Tuesday

Day 7   Sunday

Repeat Wednesday

If you wish, you can follow this diet for 30 days on a rotational basis. What follows is an option for the remaining 23 days.

Day 8   Monday

Breakfast

4 ounces red snapper, baked or broiled, lightly buttered, seasoned
      to taste
½ medium jicama, cut in slices
1 bran muffin
½ glass of prune juice

Snack

1 ounce almonds, unsalted

Lunch

Lentil soup (see recipe below)
Green salad: butter lettuce, alfalfa sprouts, olive oil dressing (all
  you wish)
Cream cheese spread on unleavened bread (matzo) square.

Snack

Popcorn, air-popped, lightly buttered

Dinner

Wedge of red cabbage with salad dressing
Medium tomato, sliced
Coffee substitute

Lentil Soup

4 cups stock or water
1 cup dried lentils, washed
1 large white onion, diced
2 stalks deep green celery,
  plus chopped tops
2 medium carrots
1 teaspoon cumin

1 teaspoon nutmeg
1 teaspoon celery seed
1 teaspoon Tamari soy
  sauce
1 teaspoon thyme
2 sprigs parsley
1 teaspoon sweet basil

Bring liquid to boil and add lentils. Reduce heat and simmer for
40 minutes, partially covered. Add rest of ingredients and simmer

for 20 minutes more. Add Tamari last to preserve its nutritional content. Remove half of soup from pan to blender and whiz for a few seconds to obtain thick, warm lentil puree. Mix back into remaining soup in pot and stir to desired consistency. Top with minced parsley.

=============== *Day 9   Tuesday* ===============

Breakfast

Two large buckwheat pancakes made with 1 egg, lightly buttered
    and served with maple syrup
Dish of fresh strawberries or equivalent frozen, unsweetened,
    with light cream, if desired
Herbal tea

Snack

1 ounce pecans

Lunch

3 ounces beef liver, broiled, lightly buttered
Green salad (all you can eat) with dressing, different from that
    used previously, and a touch of iodized sea salt
1 ounce macadamia nuts
Sparkling mineral water

Snack

4 cauliflower florets

Dinner

Irish potato, medium, baked in skin, lightly buttered, garnished
    with dill and a touch of iodized sea salt
Herbal tea

Day 10   Wednesday

Breakfast

4-ounce ground round patty, broiled
Bran muffin
6 strips green pepper
1 cup fresh blueberries or the equivalent frozen
Coffee substitute

Snack

Stick of dark green celery filled with peanut butter

Lunch

Tuna (3 ounces) salad made with Boston lettuce and sunflower
    seed dressing (all you can eat)
Slice of whole-wheat toast
Sparkling mineral water

Snack

1 ounce almonds, unsalted

Dinner

½ cucumber, sliced
Medium ear of sweet corn, lightly buttered with hint of iodized
     sea salt
Herbal tea

Day 11   Thursday

Breakfast

4-ounce lamb shoulder chop broiled
4 pieces broccoli, steamed
Slice of whole-grain rye toast, lightly buttered
Fresh peach
Coffee substitute

Snack

1 ounce walnuts

Lunch

Bowl of minestrone soup (see recipe below)
½ cup cottage cheese, sprinkled with diced chives
Fresh pear
Tangerine

Snack

1 ounce Brazil nuts

Dinner

6 asparagus spears, lightly steamed
1 cup lightly cooked beets
½ cup blackberries
Cold spring water with lemon or lime flavoring

===== *Minestrone Soup* =====

1 cup dried beans: kidney,
pinto, lima, northern, or
any other kind
4 cups water
1 large onion, chopped
2 garlic cloves, diced
2 carrots, chopped
1 celery stalk, chopped
12 ounces cabbage,
chopped

1 cup chopped spinach or
chard
1 9½-ounce can plum
tomatoes in tomato juice
1 cup whole-wheat pasta
1 teaspoon dried oregano
1 teaspoon sea salt
5 cups water (in addition
to 4 cups mentioned
above)

Soak beans overnight in 4 cups water. Cook 1 hour or until tender.
Add remaining ingredients and cook 20 minutes more or until
pasta is tender.

Serve hot, sprinkled with fresh Parmesan cheese.

===== *Day 12 Friday* =====

Repeat Monday

Day 13 Saturday

Repeat Tuesday

Day 14 Sunday

Repeat Wednesday

Day 15 Monday

Breakfast

4-ounce chicken breast, skinless, baked
½ avocado with a sprinkling of parmesan cheese
⅛ fresh pineapple in chunks
Coffee substitute

Snack

1 fig bar (health food store type)

Lunch

½ yellow squash, dusted with saffron powder and baked
Slice of barley bread toast, lightly buttered

Snack

1 ounce macadamia nuts

Dinner

Cooked millet mixed with a small, finely chopped, raw onion, 1
    clove of garlic and vegetable bacon bits
Herbal tea

═══════ *Day 16   Tuesday* ═══════

Breakfast

4-ounce halibut steak, broiled, garnished with grated parsley
1 large carrot, diced, lightly cooked, topped with thinly sliced
    scallions
1 oatmeal muffin, oven-warmed
15 fresh cherries
Coffee substitute

Snack

1 large green apple

Lunch

2 slices of lentil loaf
½ cup wax beans, steamed, with touch of butter
3 fresh plums
Sparkling mineral water

Snack

1 guava

Dinner

Artichoke, steamed, dipped in garlic-flavored olive oil
Tangerine
Herbal tea

Day 17   Wednesday

Breakfast

4-ounce veal chop, broiled
2 slices of whole-wheat toast, lightly buttered
3 fresh apricots
½ honeydew melon
1 cup soy milk

Snack

1 ounce pistachio nuts

Lunch

Wax beans and pearl onions, lighly cooked
1 cup loganberries
Glass of fresh orange juice

Snack

1 ounce hazelnuts

Dinner

½ cup chopped leek as filler in sandwich of whole-wheat bread,
    lightly buttered and sea-salted
1 medium banana
Sparkling mineral water

Day 18   Thursday

Breakfast

4 ounces sea bass, baked or broiled
Bowl of cooked brown rice, lightly buttered, dusted with carob
    powder (a chocolate substitute) with a bit of honey added
6 prunes, cooked
Coffee substitute

Snack

5 green olives

Lunch

3 ounces beef liver, broiled with sea salt and smothered with
    cooked onions
½ slice of watermelon 10″ × 1″ round
Herbal tea

Snack

1 ounce filbert nuts

Dinner

½ cup tofu flavored with tamari sauce
1 cup warm spring water flavored with 1 tablespoon honey and
    2 tablespoons carob powder

Day 19   Friday

Repeat Monday

Day 20   Saturday

Repeat Tuesday

Day 21   Sunday

Repeat Wednesday

Day 22   Monday

Breakfast

Spicy chicken: skinned breast, broiled, with a hint of butter and
   a sprinkling of paprika and sea salt
Small sweet potato, baked, with olive oil flavored to taste with
   minced garlic
Bowl of warm millet with light cream
½ pink grapefruit
Coffee substitute

Snack

3 dates

Lunch

1 cup cooked navy beans with vegetable bacon bits, flavored with
   sugar-free grape juice (a form of New Testament honey)
Wedge of raw cabbage, dipped in vinegar and lemon juice and
   lightly sea-salted
Sparkling mineral water

Snack

1 ounce cashew nuts

Dinner

Bowl of rye cereal cooked with fig fragments
Small apple
Herbal tea

Day 23   Tuesday

Breakfast

2 soft-boiled or poached eggs
Slice of whole-wheat toast, lightly buttered
Small Irish potato, baked, with dollop of sour cream, scallions,
    and sea salt added
¼ honeydew melon or equivalent in frozen melon balls
1 glass of milk

Snack

1 ounce cashew nuts

Lunch

Bowl of yellow split-pea soup (see recipe below)
1 cup high-quality, plain yogurt (Alta-Dena, if available in your
    area) blended with half a handful of fresh or frozen black-
    berries
Sparkling mineral water

Snack

Small Valencia orange

Dinner

1 cup cooked pinto beans with dash of tomato juice and, after
    cooking, mixed with shredded parsley and vegetable bacon
    bits
Glass of spring water mixed with 1 tablespoon green barley pow-
    der, juice from half a lime and teaspoon of honey

Yellow Split-Pea Soup

1 pound yellow split peas   2 stalks celery, chopped
2 carrots, diced   1 teaspoon celery salt
1 onion, chopped

Cover split peas with two inches of water. Add carrots, onions, celery and seasoning. Cook until peas are tender. Stir often. Blend for smooth soup or serve as is, with garlic toast.

Day 24　Wednesday

Breakfast

2 French lamp chops, broiled
Bowl of amaranth cereal with cherry juice
Oatmeal muffin
Glass of soy milk, thoroughly mixed with 1 tablespoon of malt
     powder and 1 tablespoon of honey
Coffee substitute

Snack

1 ounce pumpkin seeds

Lunch

½ container of sardines packed in water
1 serving of cole slaw: shredded cabbage and a dash of pineapple
     juice, juice from half a lemon and light cream
Sparkling mineral water

Snack

Popcorn, air-popped, lightly buttered

Dinner

1 ear of sweet corn, lightly buttered
2 fresh plums
Herbal tea

Day 25   Thursday

Breakfast

6-ounce filet mignon, broiled, peppered and sea-salted to taste
Slice of millet toast, lightly buttered
Strips cut from ½ green pepper
Fresh apple and celery juice (two to one ratio of apple and celery)

Snack

1 ounce pine nuts

Lunch

Three-lettuce salad with bean sprouts and vinegar and safflower
    oil dressing (all you can eat)
Fresh pear
Sparkling mineral water

Snack

Handful of raisins

Dinner

1 cup cooked millet with small date fragments, lightly buttered,
    spread with maple syrup and powdered with cinnamon
Sparkling mineral water

Day 26 Friday

Repeat Monday

Day 27 Saturday

Repeat Tuesday

Day 28 Sunday

Repeat Wednesday

═══════ *Day 29 Monday* ═══════

Breakfast

4 ounces baked turkey breast without skin
1 cup whole cranberries, cooked
Small Irish potato, with chives and light butter
Coffee substitute

Snack

1 ounce peanuts

Lunch

3-ounce salmon patty: salmon, bread crumbs, diced onion and
    garlic clove, moistened with coconut milk
Glass of coconut milk mixed with 2 tablespoons malt powder and
    1 tablespoon honey

Snack

Square of unleavened bread (matzo) lightly buttered and sea-
    salted

Dinner

Cut green beans, steamed and covered with parmesan cheese
Herbal tea

Day 30 Tuesday

Breakfast

Chicken drumstick, baked
Bowl of cooked whole rye, spiced with pimiento and onion bits
1 cup yogurt, flavored with pineapple juice
Bowl of applesauce
Herbal tea

Snack

1 ounce Brazil nuts

Lunch

Tuna salad: 3 ounces tuna, lettuce, 1 stick celery, diced, and may-
    onnaise
½ bowl of fresh red raspberries
Sparkling mineral water

Snack

Bunch of seedless grapes

Dinner

Cooked brown rice with button mushrooms and grated sharp
    cheddar cheese to be melted on concoction when returned
    to oven
Herbal tea with dash of lemon and teaspoon of honey

DIET BIBLE DIET (FOR MEN)

Approximately 1200 Calories Daily

FIRST WEEK TWO-HOUR COOKING THEME

As in the "For Women" section, this diet accents carnitine-rich foods and a one-week, or even one-month meal rotation that can be prepared in a couple of hours.

Cook 1 cup each of millet, oats, whole-rye cereal and brown rice (a week's supply). Refrigerate the cooked cereals in individual, airtight plastic containers.

Prepare 1 pound of ½-inch cubes of lamb shanks and chuck and 1 pound of smaller cubes of skinned chicken breast, as recommended in the recipes below, and refrigerate them in 4-ounce amounts in individual, airtight plastic containers.

Make lentil loaf, according to the recipe below and refrigerate in 4-ounce amounts in individual airtight plastic containers.

Fix sprout salad as directed in the recipe below and refrigerate it in a large, airtight plastic container. This salad can be stored for more than a week without deteriorating. All other items above can be frozen, if desired, and stored.

These instructions, and the recipes that follow, are also in the "For Women" section in the interest of conserving your time.

1ST WEEK   TWO-HOUR COOKING THEME (FOR MEN)

Cook 2 cups of millet and refrigerate it in a sealed plastic container. Cook 1 cup each of whole-rye cereal, oats, and brown rice and refrigerate them in individual plastic containers.

Prepare the following recipes:

══ King David's Lamb with Lentils ══

1 pound lamb shank	Dash cayenne
garlic	2½ cups dried lentils
3 tablespoons olive oil	¼ cup chopped parsley
1 onion, minced	4 leeks, minced
½ teaspoon rosemary	

Cut lamb into ½-inch cubes. Insert a garlic sliver into each cube and brown them in 2 tablespoons oil, then add ½ cup water and simmer, turning cubes often and adding more water, if necessary, until meat is tender.

Saute onion in 1 tablespoon oil until translucent. Add rosemary and cayenne and bring to boil. Add washed and strained lentils and 3 cups water. Return to boil, cover and simmer 45 minutes to 1 hour. Stir parsley and scallions into cooked lentils. Divide lentil mixture into 4 servings and top them with equal amounts of lamb cubes. Refrigerate each serving in a plastic container until ready to serve.

Bible Beef

1 pound lean chuck	½ teaspoon marjoram
1 medium-size onion	¼ teaspoon sea salt
Clove garlic	

Place 1 pound chuck cut into ½-inch cubes in frying pan. Sprinkle with marjoram and sea salt. Add 1 cup water to cover bottom of pan. Dice onions and garlic and add to chuck. Simmer, stirring often and adding water as necessary, until tender. Refrigerate ¼-pound servings in individual sealed plastic containers and refrigerate until required for rewarming.

Chicken and Leeks

1 pound boned and skinned chicken breasts	¼ teaspoon sea salt
¼ pound leeks	Dash of paprika

Cut chicken into ½-inch cubes and place in frying pan. Add salt, paprika and chopped leeks to chicken and cover bottom of pan with ¼-inch spring water.

Stew chicken, turning often and adding water, if necessary. When tender, refrigerate in sealed plastic container.

Lentil Loaf

2 cups lentils	1 clove garlic, crushed
1 teaspoon sea salt	2 medium peeled, seeded
2 tablespoons olive oil	and chopped tomatoes
1 medium onion, minced	2 eggs, beaten

Cook lentils in 4-½ cups water with salt for 35 minutes or until done. Heat oven to 350°F.

Heat olive oil and saute onion until transparent. Add onion and oil to cooked lentils. Add all other ingredients. Add lentil mixture to oiled loaf pan, pat with fork to shape well, and bake for 45 minutes. Good hot or cold.

Refrigerate in airtight containers until ready for use.

Sprout Salad

This salad is virtually nonallergenic and can be repeated. Stored in an airtight plastic container, sprout salad keeps for more than a week without deteriorating, as I have learned. Here is the recipe:

2 pounds bean sprouts	2 bunches seedless red or
2 red apples	green grapes
2 cups seedless raisins	1 stalk celery
1 dozen green onions	1 pound pine nuts or
	walnuts
	2 bunches cilantro

Cut apples, onions, celery and cilantro into fragments. Good with or without dressing.

First Theme Week Diet (for Men):

Day 1   Monday

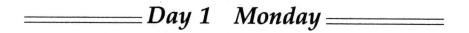

Breakfast

4 ounces cooked lamb shank cubes with lentils, heated (recipe
    above)
1 cup fresh carrot juice or 3 small scrubbed carrots
2 slices of whole grain wheat bread, lightly buttered
Glass of whole milk

Snack

1 large winesap apple

Lunch:

½ container of sardines
Slice of lentil loaf, warmed
Sprout salad (all you wish) with dressing of choice
Small cluster (12) of seedless grapes
Sparkling mineral water

Snack

Large banana

Dinner

Cup of cucumber and celery juice made in blender
Bowl of cold millet flavored with ¼-cup unsweetened pineapple juice
Camomile tea
(This high carbohydrate meal may promote sound sleep.)

=============== *Day 2   Tuesday* ===============

Breakfast

4 ounces beef stew, on base of cooked, rewarmed rye cereal
2 bran muffins
Sprout salad with a dressing different from yesterday's
6 cooked prunes
Coffee substitute

Snack

10 fresh strawberries in season or same amount unsweetened fresh frozen.

Lunch

2 hard-boiled eggs
Slice whole-rye toast
5 green olives
Sparkling mineral water

Snack

1 ounce sunflower seeds

Dinner

Bowl of warmed brown rice, lightly buttered, spread with unfiltered, unprocessed honey and snowed over with cinnamon.
Red Zinger tea

════════ Day 3   Wednesday ════════

Breakfast

1 cup warmed diced chicken and leeks (4 ounces) served on a bed of cooked oats with a dash of olive oil, if desired.
2 slices of barley bread toast
6 dates
Herbal tea

Snack

½ cup blueberries in season or same amount unsweetened fresh frozen

Lunch

Sprout salad (all you can eat) with a dressing different from previous day's
Medium baked sweet potato, lightly buttered
Sparkling mineral water

Snack

2 ounces pumpkin seeds

Dinner

1 square of unleavened bread (matzo) lightly buttered
½ fresh cantaloupe or the same amount of fresh frozen melon
    balls
Herbal tea

Day 4   Thursday

Breakfast

4 ounces salmon steak, broiled, garnished with capers
Dish of steamed zucchini, lightly buttered
Bowl of boysenberries with a dash of coffee cream
½ pink grapefruit

Snack

2 ounces cashew nuts

Lunch

Sprout salad (all you can eat) with vinaigrette dressing
1 orange

Snack

2 ounces walnut meats

Dinner

Bowl of amaranth cereal with cherry juice
Glass of sparkling mineral water, with squeezing of ½ lime and
    1 tablespoon honey

Day 5 Friday

Repeat Monday

Day 6 Saturday

Repeat Tuesday

Day 7 Sunday

Repeat Wednesday

For those who wish, this diet can be followed for 30 days on a rotational basis. What follows is an option for the remaining 23 days.

Day 8   Monday

Breakfast

4 ounces red snapper, baked or broiled
Bowl of cooked millet with light cream
Bowl of steamed, yellow squash
10 pods of fresh peas or 3 tablespoons frozen peas
Glass of milk (certified raw, if available)

Snack

1 ounce almonds, unsalted

Lunch

Lentil soup (see recipe below)
Bran muffin, lightly buttered
Green salad: butter lettuce, alfalfa sprouts, olive oil dressing (all
    you wish)
1-inch round of watermelon
Glass of sparkling mineral water mixed with 2 tablespoons carob
    powder and 1 tablespoon honey

Snack

Popcorn, air-popped, lightly buttered

Dinner

Wedge of red cabbage (with salad dressing, if desired)
½ medium tomato, sliced
Coffee substitute

Lentil Soup

4 cups stock or water
1 cup dried lentils, washed
1 large white onion, diced
2 stalks deep green celery,
    plus chopped tops
2 medium carrots
1 teaspoon cumin

1 teaspoon nutmeg
1 teaspoon celery seed
1 tablespoon Tamari soy
    sauce
1 teaspoon thyme
2 sprigs parsley
1 teaspoon sweet basil

Bring liquid to boil and add lentils. Reduce heat and simmer for 40 minutes, partially covered. Add rest of ingredients and simmer for 20 minutes more. Add Tamari last to preserve its nutritional content. Remove half of soup from pan to blender and whiz for a few seconds to obtain thick, warm, lentil puree. Mix back into remaining soup in pot and stir to desired consistency. Top with minced parsley.

Day 9   Tuesday

Breakfast

4 large buckwheat pancakes made with 2 eggs, lightly buttered
    and served with maple syrup
½ medium jicama, sliced
Dish of fresh strawberries or equivalent amount frozen, unsweet-
    ened
Herbal tea

Snack

2 ounces pecans

Lunch

Medium Irish potato, baked in skin, lightly buttered, garnished
    with dill and iodized salt
1 medium banana

Snack

2 ounces Brazil nuts

Dinner

Green salad (all you can eat) with dressing of choice different
    from previous day's and a touch of iodized sea salt
Small bowl of cooked turnips, lightly dusted with cayenne and
    sea salt
Glass of buttermilk

═══ Day 10 Wednesday ═══

Breakfast

4-ounce ground round patty, broiled
2 slices of whole-wheat toast
½ green pepper in strips
Dish of fresh blueberries or equivalent amount frozen
Coffee substitute

Snack

Stick of dark green celery filled with peanut butter

Lunch

Tuna (4 ounces) salad made with Boston lettuce and sunflower
    seed dressing (all you can eat)
Medium tangerine
3 ounces green beans, steamed, topped with vegetable bacon bits
Sparkling mineral water

Snack

1 ounce almonds, unsalted

Dinner

½ cucumber, sliced
Medium ear of sweet corn, lightly buttered, with a hint of iodized
    sea salt
½ glass of prune juice

Day 11   Thursday

Breakfast

4-ounce lamb shoulder chop, broiled
6 pieces broccoli, steamed
2 slices of whole-grain rye toast, lightly buttered
Bowl of loganberries
Coffee substitute

Snack

1 ounce walnut meats

Lunch

Bowl of minestrone soup (see recipe below)
1 Fresh pear

Snack

1 ounce Brazil nuts

Dinner

4 asparagus spears, steamed
Dish of rutabaga, lightly steamed, with pat of butter
Cold spring water with lemon or lime flavoring

═══ Minestrone Soup ═══

1 cup dried beans: kidney, pinto, lima, northern, or any other kind	1 cup chopped spinach or chard
4 cups water	1 9-½-ounce can plum tomatoes in tomato juice
1 large onion, chopped	1 cup whole-wheat pasta
2 garlic cloves, diced	1 teaspoon dried oregano
2 carrots, chopped	1 teaspoon sea salt
1 celery stalk, chopped	5 cups water (in addition to 4 cups mentioned above)
12 ounce cabbage, chopped	

Soak beans overnight in 4 cups water. Cook 1 hour or until tender. Add remaining ingredients and cook 20 minutes more, or until pasta is tender.

Serve hot, sprinkled with fresh parmesan cheese.

Day 12   Friday

Repeat Monday

Day 13   Saturday

Repeat Tuesday

Day 14 Sunday

Repeat Wednesday

Day 15   Monday

Breakfast

4-ounce chicken breast, skinless, baked
½ avocado with sprinkling of shredded cheddar cheese
¼ fresh pineapple in chunks
3 unsulphured dates
Coffee substitute

Snack

3 fig bars (health food store type)

Lunch

Cooked millet mixed with small, finely chopped raw onion, 1
   clove finely chopped garlic and vegetable bacon bits
½ cantaloupe or equivalent in frozen cantaloupe balls

Snack

1 ounce peanuts

Dinner

½ yellow squash, dusted with saffron powder and baked
Large orange
Herbal tea

══════ *Day 16   Tuesday* ══════

Breakfast

4-ounce halibut steak, broiled, garnished with grated parsley
Large carrot sliced and lightly cooked, topped with thinly sliced
   scallions
2 bran muffins, oven-warmed
2 fresh plums
bowl of cooked brown rice, lightly buttered with maple syrup and
   sprinkling of cinnamon
Coffee substitute

Snack

1 large Granny Smith apple

Lunch

Bowl of iced cucumber soup (see recipe below)
½ cup wax beans, steamed, with touch of butter
Sparkling mineral water

Snack

1 large, fresh peach

Dinner

Artichoke, steamed, each helping dipped in garlic-flavored olive
   oil
12 seedless grapes
Herbal tea

Iced Cucumber Soup

2 cucumbers	1 tablespoon minced
4 scallions	parsley
1 tablespoon vegetable oil	1 cup sour cream or same
3 cups vegetable cooking	amount of yogurt
water	Sea salt to taste

Dice 1 cucumber. Chop scallions. Saute scallions in oil until translucent. Add cucumber and stir briefly. Add vegetable water and simmer, covered, 10 minutes or until cucumber is very soft. Add parsley to broth and puree mixture in blender. Seed remaining cucumber and grate into puree. Let soup cool to lukewarm. Stir in sour cream or yogurt and salt to taste. Chill. Serve cold.

═══════ *Day 17 Wednesday* ═══════

Breakfast

4-ounce veal chop broiled
2 slices of toasted barley bread, lightly buttered
½ large tomato, sliced and garnished with dill
3 fresh apricots
Coffee substitute

Snack

1 ounce pistachio nuts

Lunch

String beans and small pearl onions, lightly cooked
½ large tomato, sliced and garnished with dill
5 radishes
½ glass of cranberry juice

Snack

1 ounce hazelnuts

Dinner

½ cup chopped leek as filler in sandwich of oatmeal bread, lightly
    buttered and sea-salted
10 fresh cherries or fresh frozen equivalent
Sparkling mineral water

Day 18   Thursday

Breakfast

4 ounces sea bass, baked or broiled
½ cup cooked spinach, topped with grated cheddar cheese
2 buckwheat mufflins, warmed
6 prunes, cooked
Coffee substitute

Snack

4 green olives

Lunch

3 ounces beef liver, broiled, with hint of sea salt and black pepper,
     smothered with cooked onions
⅓ cup cooked beets
Slice of watermelon, 1 inch thick
Herbal tea

Snack

1 ounce filbert nuts

Dinner

⅔ cup tofu flavored with tamari sauce
Warm bottled spring water flavored with 2 heaping tablespoons
     carob powder and 1 tablespoon honey, mixed well

Day 19 Friday

Repeat Monday

Day 20 Saturday

Repeat Tuesday

Day 21 Sunday

Repeat Wednesday

Day 22 Monday

Breakfast

Spicy chicken: skinned breast, baked with a hint of butter and a
sprinkling of paprika and sea salt
Medium yam, baked, flavored with olive oil and minced garlic to
taste
2 oatmeal muffins
½ pink grapefrut
Coffee substitute

Snack

Medium banana

Lunch

1 cup cooked navy beans, flavored with sugar-free grape juice (a
   form of New Testament honey) and vegetable bacon bits
Wedge of raw cabbage, dipped in vinegar and lemon juice and
   lightly sea-salted
Tangerine

Snack

1 ounce cashew nuts

Dinner

1 cup cooked rye cereal with small fig fragments
Iceberg lettuce and alfalfa sprout salad with sunflower oil dressing
Herbal tea

Day 23 Tuesday

Breakfast

2 soft-boiled or poached eggs
Medium Irish potato, baked, with dollop sour cream, scallions
   and light sea salt added
2 slices of whole-wheat toast, lightly buttered
½ honeydew melon or equivalent in frozen melon balls
Coffee substitute

Snack

1 ounce almonds

Lunch

Bowl of yellow split-pea soup (see recipe below)
1 cup high-quality, plain yogurt (such as Alta-Dena, if available
    in your area) blended with handful of fresh or frozen black-
    berries
Sparkling mineral water

Snack

Valencia orange

Dinner

½ cup cooked navy beans mixed with ¼ cup tomato juice and,
    after warming, ⅓ cup shredded parsley and same amount
    of vegetable bacon bits
Glass of spring water, mixed well with 1 tablespoon green barley
    powder, juice from ½ lime and 1 tablespoon honey

Yellow Split-Pea Soup

1 pound yellow split peas	2 stalks celery, chopped
2 carrots, diced	1 teaspoon celery salt
1 onion, chopped	

Cover split peas with 2 inches of water. Add carrots, onions, celery and seasoning. Cook until peas are tender, stirring often. Blend for smooth soup or serve as is, with garlic toast.

Day 24 Wednesday

Breakfast

2 French lamb chops, broiled
2 slices of whole-rye toast
Bowl of amaranth cereal flavored with cherry juice
½ guava fruit
Coffee substitute

Snack

1 ounce pumpkin seeds

Lunch

½ container of sardines packed in water
Serving of cole slaw: shredded cabbage and a blend of 1 dash
    pineapple juice, juice from ½ lemon and a small amount of
    light cream

Snack

½ cucumber
1 ounce sunflower seeds

Dinner

1 ear of sweet corn, lightly buttered and sea-salted
Dish of cooked, diced rutabagas and turnips, with sprinkling of
    saffron
Herbal tea

Day 25   Thursday

Breakfast

6-ounce filet mignon broiled, salted and peppered to taste
1 slice of oatmeal bread toast
½ green pepper, cut in strips
Glass of fresh apple and celery juice (2 to 1 ratio of apple and
    celery)

Snack

1 ounce piñon nuts

Lunch

½ cup cooked lima beans with sliced carrots and pearl onions
Three-lettuce salad with alfalfa sprouts and vinegar and safflower
    oil dressing (all you can eat)
Fresh pear
Sparkling mineral water

Snack

Handful of raisins

Dinner

½ medium jicama in slices
1 cup cooked millet with small date fragments, lightly buttered,
    spread with honey and powdered with cinnamon
Sparkling mineral water

Day 26 Friday

Same as Monday

Day 27 Saturday

Same as Tuesday

Day 28 Sunday

Same as Wednesday

Day 29 Monday

Breakfast

4 ounces baked turkey breast without skin
1 cup cooked cranberries
2 ounces cheddar cheese
2 slices of barley bread toast
Coffee substitute

Snack

1 ounce peanuts

Lunch

4-ounce salmon patty: salmon, bread crumbs, diced onion and
garlic clove, moistened with coconut milk
Glass of coconut milk milkshake, flavored with 2 tablespoons
carob powder and 1 tablespoon honey.

Snack

Unleavened bread (matzo) lightly buttered and sea-salted

Dinner

Bowl of lentil soup (See recipe under Day 8)
1 cup cut green beans, steamed, covered with parmesan cheese
Herbal tea

━━━━━ Day 30   Tuesday ━━━━━

Breakfast

Chicken drumstick, baked
Bowl of applesauce
2 slices of corn bread
Bowl of cooked whole-grain wheat, spiced with pimento and on-
ion bits
Herbal tea

Snack

1 ounce macadamia nuts

Lunch

Tuna salad (lettuce, tuna, diced celery and mayonnaise)
Bowl of fresh or frozen red raspberries
Sparkling mineral water

Snack

Pineapple slice, fresh

Dinner

Brown rice cooked with button mushrooms (1 cup cooked), with
grated sharp cheddar cheese melted into concoction when
returned to oven
Herbal tea with dash of lemon and teaspoon of honey